HOW TO EMBRACE YOUR **INNER**

Hotness

An **INSIDE**-Out Approach
to a Lasting
makeover

Leta Greene

This is a work of creative nonfiction. The events herein are portrayed to the best of the author's memory. While all the stories in this book are true, some names and identifying details may have been changed to protect the privacy of the people involved.

Editorial work by Eschler Editing
Cover design by Kent Hepworth
Interior design and layout by Ben Welch

Printed by Stonebridge Printing

Printed in the United States of America
10 9 8 7 6 5 4
ISBN 978-0-9895523-2-5

You can also buy Leta's audiobook at http://letagreene.biz/book/

DEDICATION

*To the man who loves me the most and
to the children with whom God has blessed us.*

Table of Contents

Now That You're Hot
Finding or Rediscovering Your Perfect Match

Happily Ever After Is a Choice?
How to Keep the New You Growing Hotter Every Day

Introduction

---- ✍ ----

WE'RE ALL UGLY DUCKLINGS

Beauty. We all want it. Our toes curl with excitement the first time a boy tells us we're beautiful. But it sure seems easier said than done. The standard of "beauty" is held so far out of our reach that we spend amazing sums of money on potions and lotions to maintain or achieve what we are told is beautiful. The ancient cave woman had it so good: no mirrors. And no fashion models in the latest cave-wear showing her just how outdated she was—SO last year. Her value was based on making cave babies and staying alive. (Well, maybe she didn't have it *that* good.)

As a young teen, I was a very fashionable cave girl. No, not because I'm that old. Because I didn't have all of my teeth. (More about that later!) Therefore I was pretty sure that I wasn't beautiful. Think about it. Wouldn't you agree that supermodels have all their teeth? Ever seen an icon of beauty without her pearly whites? All magazine-worthy smiles come in airbrushed perfection, all teeth accounted for. How about a prom queen? A beauty pageant contestant? Yes, all of them have teeth. Recognize a pattern here?

I saw that pattern, big as life. Beautiful equals a perfect dental display of pearly whites. But I didn't have one. I sported a *big gap*. Right at the front of my mouth. I tried hard not to smile. Not to let others see. I held my hand to my mouth to cover what wasn't there, but hiding the facts from the public only went so far. Every time I looked in the mirror I saw what was missing, and it reminded me I was not a beauty. I knew that when my Prince Charming arrived to swoop me into his arms, I would smile, and . . . *whoa* . . . he would drop me unceremoniously on my toothless peasant bottom and ride off on his gallant steed in search of a maiden worthy of his love—one with ALL of her teeth.

And so it was. Every time I looked in the mirror, I saw it. That toothless gap solidified my lack of worth, the impossibility of future happiness, and my shortness of beauty. I wasn't stupid. I knew that joy, beauty, and fulfilled dreams belonged only to *other* women—the perfect ones.

Is that how it is? (If you're nodding your head, stop it!) My response to those ideas has changed a lot since I became a makeup artist and image consultant. How weird is that? These days I just roll my eyes and ask, "*Really?*" But that is what Hollywood, the diet industry, the fashion industry, and so many more are still trying to sells us.

It's peddled by Madison Avenue. By countless magazine covers. By models on whom every last trace of wrinkles, cellulite, and zits—not to mention imperfect teeth—has been relentlessly airbrushed into oblivion. By ninety-pound thirteen-year-olds held up as examples of what we should look like—and shame on us if we don't. And they are all lies. Very pretty lies, to be sure, but lies that come with a devastating collateral of crushed confidence and trampled self-worth.

We see symptoms of our buy-in all around us. It's manifest by fourth graders going on crash diets to get thinner. In the growing epidemic of often dangerous, unnecessary plastic surgery. In Botox injections and laser facials and chemical peels. In the over-sexualization of women in general—and of very young girls and young women in particular—all because they believe that the only valuable thing they have to offer is sex appeal.

What's most shocking is that *everybody* has some level of buy-in, even if they meet the standard. I've seen it from models to attractive supermoms (who pass it on generationally without even realizing it). Every woman I've talked to thinks she just doesn't measure up. Even putting aside that our culture spawns a demolition of women's *inner* worth, much of our potential outer beauty is also destroyed by the can't-measure-up opt-in. After all, we project what we feel inside. Sooner or later, even the beauty queen loses attention because she's just not pretty to be with.

Here's the problem: We think we are ugly when in reality we are creatures of immeasurable beauty. We've accepted the world's definition of *beauty* without seeing things as they really are. We don't have a *beauty* problem. We have a *vision* problem. We need to learn to see with better eyes—with the eyes of the heart and the spirit, not with physical eyes that have been brainwashed by society and by the faulty vision of those around us. We need to get true twenty-twenty beauty vision.

Seeing things as they really are will likely cause us to look at beauty in a whole new way. Beauty isn't an arbitrary value society assigns us but rather something deep and inherent in our souls. We are beautiful because we are unique in all the universe. Becoming gorgeous is about recognizing yourself regardless of the package and wrapping you come in at any given time.

The story of becoming beautiful is not about the ugly duckling becoming a swan; it is about the duckling realizing that it was a swan all along. The ugly duckling failed to radiate what it really was because it had *bought in*. It was teased for not fitting in, and it took the word of the other birds and just accepted that it was subpar. We're just like that little ugly duckling, because even though we are born with infinite potential and can be gorgeous inside and out, somehow we become convinced that we are misfits—that we are different and that different is bad.

We are told that to be beautiful we need to have an outer transformation similar to that duckling finally *looking* like a swan. The other ducks teased the misplaced swan, but if human/swan nature is any indication, it probably also got teased once it was with the swans. Maybe it also got teased for spending its childhood among the ducks, and on and on. We get tripped up by focusing on all the differences, be we duck, swan, or human. The differences are what make us unique—and later, we might find that instead of being "wrong," those are the things we actually love about our appearance. (The redhead who is called "carrot top" later finds that she loves her hair!)

When I was younger, I had my own perspective of what was right, and because I didn't conform to that perspective, I didn't fit in. But in life, *all of us* tend to feel we are ugly ducklings in one way or another. Don't believe me yet? I *know* it's true. In my business, I've talked to women from every slice of life who felt like that. Plenty of women who were "cheerleaders," the so-called "popular girls," models, trophy wives, athletes, dancers, yoga and Pilates divas, and all the rest. They all felt the same way—they believed they weren't enough. Not popular enough. Not slim enough. Not good enough. Not pretty enough.

What does it mean to be "enough"? Is our goal to be like everyone else? It shouldn't be, because we are each a unique and special canvas created by a loving God for a particular purpose—our own, not someone else's. Realizing our purpose is not about a fundamental transformation of our physical features; it is about a fundamental transformation of what we feel about our value.

And that brings us to why I finally wrote this book. I had my fundamental transformation, and the freedom I found to be hot convinced me everyone needs to own their hotness too.

Remember my toothless childhood? Well, I finally got that fixed. But the universe is full of practical jokes, and I am now toothless again—that's right, as an image consultant. You're probably wondering how that affects my job. I'll share the details to make my point about transformations.

So to start, I was rear-ended by a texting teenage driver. Small time-out for a public service announcement: Texting + driving = bad.

My kids were okay, but I had whiplash, and my bumper was sad. I didn't realize anything was wrong at first, but within days my mouth really started to hurt. So I went to the dentist.

Unbelievably, the accident had compromised one of my fake teeth, and an infection had spread through my jaw. The tooth would have to be removed, and the bone needed time to heal before an implant could be put in. In the meantime, just to preserve any sort of normalcy, I was fitted with a retainer that had a tooth on it.

Things are so much different now than when I was a kid. True, I again have a big gap where that tooth is supposed to be. That absolutely devastated me when I was a kid. But now, with the perspective of twenty years, I have decided to make that missing tooth work for me. I am not supposed to eat with the retainer (and, hence, the tooth) in my mouth. So whenever I sit down to eat—including at fancy dinners with my hubby's work, at conferences where I am speaking, at networking meetings, out with friends, at church dinners—the tooth gets tucked in a napkin. It's kinda fun. I can pretend that it popped out as I start looking frantically around at other plates, as though I might find it sitting atop someone else's broccoli. Or I can simply announce it to the table, which is what my etiquette-coach friend suggested, to put everyone at ease. Talk about an icebreaker!

As part of my campaign to make the tooth work *for* me, I learned how to wiggle it, delighting small children and making adults laugh out loud! They still notice; they still stare. But now I don't look away ashamed; now I make a goofy face, and we all laugh together. We are bonded. Sometimes I pop in my retainer and wiggle the tooth for whoever I catch looking. When asked how I handle it, I tell them that "any skill worth having is worth practicing!" (The skill being self-esteem. That's right, ladies. You have to develop it through working on your paradigm shifts.)

Making lemonade from lemons is easy—all you have to do is add water and sugar. But is it possible to make lemonade with a really sour lemon? That's an art form, and it usually only happens once you decide to find a purpose for whatever life gives you. For instance, did you know that even rotten lemons are a good cleaner for your disposal? They are still useful as sanitizer in your kitchen too. Just because something isn't exactly perfect doesn't mean it can't be useful. And when something of yours isn't perfect, well, that's what makes you special and you can use it to be even hotter—more confident and radiant inside and out. Just like my tooth. I'm not sure I really want to get it fixed! I love using it in my speaking, I love how it instantly relieves the get-to-know-you tension at dinner parties, I love that it makes me different—after all, most beauty experts have all of their teeth! Why be like everyone else? I like being different!

So that's it: I have a big, obvious gap in the front of my mouth. When I was a kid, a teen, and twenty years old, I couldn't' take it. But at forty, it's a whole different story. I am okay with what is missing, because what is different gives me perspective, makes me unique, and shows me how amazing we all are! I'm not trying to be "perfect." I'm happy with being me. (And I can't wait to dress up for Halloween—I'm seriously so excited! I am going to be "the glam pirate." And yes, I will take pictures.)

So to wrap up, this book tells part of the story of how I became the woman who finally figured out what transformation means, and how it affects what we are inside and out. And thus it contains the true secrets to beauty that I learned along the way—how to embrace inner hotness and transform *yourself* from the inside out. And yes, there are even secrets to claiming your own outer beauty that I'm giving up in this little book as well. But as you'll see, they won't provide the lasting makeover you're looking for without the inner change. These beauty secrets are universal principles that apply to everyone, not just me. These principles, which I have shared with both clients and friends, have helped them transform the way they see themselves, just as they once helped me do the same. They've been tested and proven, not only on my first guinea pig—myself—but on hundreds more.

After I give a speech or do coaching on this subject, I'm typically asked, "Where can I learn more?" Women want this coaching one-on-one because they get a taste of how it can change their lives. Unfortunately, there's only so much of me to go around. My kids need to see me on a regular basis; they think I'm their mom! My husband seems to like me too. As nice as it would be to sit down with each of you and share some girlfriend time, I just can't. But that's why I finally put this book together—it's my way of helping you learn more. Think of it as a map for navigating to a peak from which you can really get some perspective and see yourself for what you really are: an amazing, wonderful, wise, gorgeous woman. Trust me, you'll see the changes inside *and* out. Enjoy learning to embrace your inner hotness!

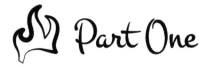 Part One

AN INSIDE-OUT MAKEOVER
BUILDING YOUR HOTNESS FROM THE GROUND UP

Beauty is what you feel about yourself,
not about what you see in the mirror.

—Unknown

Chapter One

FINDING THE INNER YOU
SHE'S WORTH GETTING TO KNOW

I WAS BORN AN HEIRESS—to a trucking company. My limo was a big rig. My fashion could be found on the cover of *Outdoor Life*—blue jeans and flannel. I could grease an axle, bench press 165 pounds, and beat all the boys at arm wrestling. Needless to say, I was not the cute girl, but I knew I could beat her up if I wanted. Add to that the fact that I had my dad's chin—a *manly* chin—and you already had a recipe for a beauty disaster. As if that weren't bad enough, *then* I had the accident.

They've repaved the road where that accident happened; it looks less menacing now. I remember it being much steeper. The gravel that made my bicycle tire skid out of control is gone. What were once foothill grasses are now trimmed flowerbeds, making the hill seem less legendary. But back then it was the stage, and I was Evel Knievel on a pink bike with a banana seat and tassels.

I started at the top, wind blowing through my hair, feeling alive and free. As my speed picked up, I wanted even more speed—until the handlebars started shaking, that is. I was going so fast that the amazing piece of pink-tasseled engineering I was riding wasn't up for the task. I lost control, hit a curb, and began to fly. The bike remained where it was.

Flying solo for thirty feet and landing on a combo of my face and arms made me pass out. When I finally woke up after lying on the side of the road for a time, I wished I'd had an audience. Not that I wanted people to see my spectacular screw-up, but so someone could have gone and gotten my mom.

My daredevil routine didn't make me famous, but it gave me several souvenirs: a long, deep gash on my chin that exposed my bone; several facial lacerations; gravel and dirt embedded in the flesh of my face and arms; and three missing front teeth. My parents sacrificed to put my chin back together, but the scar remained long after the stitches were gone. My smile, when I dared to share it, was fitted with temporary caps—until the day I left my retainer on the lunch tray.

Why do I share all of this? To give you a picture of where I was so that if you see even a sliver of yourself in my journey and feel as I did, you can know there is hope. I am no longer the girl that the boys wanted to be "just friends" with. I am no longer the sad little girl filled with insecurities. I am a chickybabe. I have my own unique *hotness*, and so do you. It is simply a matter of knowing where—and through what eyes—to look.

Children have a perfect blend of adventure and willingness to try. That is what makes childhood so magical; we don't see our limitations. This is manifest by the fact that as young children we know that we will be astronauts, the president, and beauty pageant queens. Most little girls don't look in the mirror and see themselves as ugly. I remember my daughter at six dancing in front of the mirror, saying how cute she was. My mother says that I did similar things. Like the poem says, little girls really are sugar and spice and everything nice. So what changes? What robs us of this fundamental truth?

Time.

As we get older, we start comparing ourselves to others. We begin to notice differences and assume that those differences make us wrong, flawed, and ugly. We all see those flawed, ugly differences, whether they consist of a gigantic white scar across our chin or a smattering of freckles that some neighborhood boy chooses to make fun of. Maybe we see our teeth as being crooked or our eyes as being too close together. We look in the mirror and know that no one else on Earth has a nose this big or hair this frizzy. Whatever our flaws, we will find them because we have been trained by society to search them out. We feel alone because some invisible boogie man is trying to make us think we are the only one with all these flaws. But we're not.

Beauty hang-ups are the adult version of the boogie man. They encompass all those sinister, lurking ideas about which parts of ourselves are less than beautiful—the parts we dwell on, the parts we point out to others, the parts we shamefully attempt to hide by altering our very approach to life. We change how we dress or do our makeup, we put on an air of confidence, and we carefully choose with whom we risk sharing ourselves and our gifts. If we could just fix all of these less-than-beautiful things, there'd be nothing left to run from, cover up, or hide from, right?

Wrong. No matter how "perfect" we become on the outside, our beauty boogie men will still be there—hiding in the closet of our mind, waiting to jump out and scare us anytime we let our guard down and start to feel safe. These boogie men are everywhere. They come from our families, our culture, and even our own self-talk. We can't escape them.

I learned this rather painfully. When I was barely fifteen, Mom announced we were moving. To a town named Blanding! BLANDing? I didn't want to move. We had lived in the same house for most of my life. I had gone to the same school. I knew who the mean kids were. I knew where I could walk to escape being mocked. I knew the boundaries of safety in my world, but in a new place? All I would have was my family. I didn't feel super comforted by this. In fact, I already had poor self-esteem due to some thoughtless family members.

When it comes right down to it, all any of us has is our family, at least during those early, formative years. We learn to walk and talk in our families. We also learn how to think, and our experiences in our families are the foundation for our thoughts about everything—but especially about ourselves.

And at that point in my life, facing a move and knowing that my only "safety" would be my family, I was in trouble. Each family has its own language—the way they speak, the rules they all know, and the way they agree to operate in that space. I had a problem: The space I occupied didn't fit me. This happens to a lot of people; some rebel, some learn to work within the group, and some learn to define a new truth or a new space. And some just stay trapped in the space that others have defined for them because the boogie men inside their heads tell them that no other place will accept them either.

That was me. I was trapped. Lots of factors contributed to that, but I'll share just one: my grandmother. She used to say that "no one is completely useless, if only to serve as a hideous example." There's great irony in that statement, considering her example. She is actually the source of my beauty genius—but only because after many years I was able to harness what I learned from her to empower me rather than to beat me down. She repeatedly told me how unattractive I was, how "unfortunate, really," and how heavy I was. She even discouraged me from eating at family functions with her withering, disapproving looks. My grandmother's expectations for me were low—very low. And I believed her. I didn't think I was worth much. I let her and others hurt me.

The point here is not that my grandmother was mean or that she said stupid things to me. (I have forgiven her and she did apologize decades later.) The point—and the problem—was that *I believed her.* I took those words to heart. It made an odd sort of sense to me when my grandfather told me I was too heavy in comparison to my cousins, or that it would be a bad investment to help me with college like he did my sister and my cousins. I was the ugly step-cousin. At family gatherings, I did the dishes. I didn't expect privileges, and I didn't get them.

I had learned the language of my family. I looked in the mirror and I saw an awkward, big, missing-toothed, scarred-chin castoff. I believed that life would not hold for me the kinds of things it held for others. And life reinforced that view. Here is the bitter truth: When we believe something so clearly, everything around us will make it happen. The comments, comparisons, and offenses to my soul continued because I accepted them. It hurt as a child to be placed aside, but as an adult I had to really question if I was truly not worth the dollars or personal interest that was being withheld.

Why share all of this? My childhood is filled with painful experiences. The vibe I sent out was clearly read by more than just those fluent in our family culture; even people outside our family got the message. I was hurt in terrible ways because I didn't value myself. In the Bible it talks about loving thyself. I didn't know what that meant. What I felt in my family, I projected to the world.

Maybe you're lucky and your family wasn't like mine. Does that mean you were out of the woods? No! Even if we reach kindergarten without too many family-inflicted scars, our culture is sure to step up and take care of the job.

Here's why: Our culture is largely determined by the economic interests of people we will probably never meet. We can't control the media images and ideas about beauty that assault us from the time we're old enough to notice the TV or billboards. The power brokers in the beauty and weight-loss industries who are concerned only with their financial statements will continue to airbrush fabulously figured women until their likenesses go way beyond perfection. Women of all ages will forever be bombarded with an unobtainable, shallow ideal of what will make them loved. Sex sells, and it isn't likely to stop selling anytime in the near future. The intent of these images is to amplify our insecurities in order to sell us stuff.

Hand in hand with the media are well-meaning (or mean-meaning) people we *do* meet who hardly know what kind of pain they're causing. Classmates, "friends," stinky boys, strangers, and others often act out of their own pain or their own beauty brainwashing to inflict scars that can stay with us for life.

Those things had happened to me. I had suffered from plenty of teasing as a child. I was determined not to suffer as a teen. So when my mother announced that we were moving, I was determined that Blanding would be a turning point in my life.

The first day at my new school I mustered up an incredible show of confidence. I stood up straight. I tried to look people in the eye when I talked to them. I tried not to be a dork. Things were going pretty well until I was asked to introduce myself in front of the class. Unfortunately, sometimes kids will be kids. When I stood in front of that class and said my name, everyone laughed. They didn't just laugh in that class; they pointed and laughed at me all day. I realized why—I really *was* that ugly and dumb. The kids in Blanding hadn't been gradually broken into what was so absolutely awful about me like they had been back home. In Blanding, they got the shock diet: they saw me for exactly what I was. And they laughed, pointing at me and saying my name.

On the way home that day, feeling completely broken, I said what they said, mumbling my name. I said it again. Suddenly, I heard my name in a new way—the same way those kids had heard it: "Lead-'em-On." Great. *A streetwalker name!* Even my name mocked me. And I listened. I got the message. I'd tried to hide my dorkiness, and I'd failed. With their version of my name, they had something concrete to make fun of. But their words were not nearly as damaging as the ones I began saying to myself.

Our brains are very clever. They want to save us time figuring things out. The brain makes connections between ideas so we can figure things out more quickly as time goes on. Two plus two was complicated at first; with repetition, though, we don't even have to think about it. We know the answer. Pathways in the brain are formed by repetition. According to the Practical Memory Institute, whatever we tell the brain repeatedly becomes ingrained and creates connections between the synapses. When we focus on these thoughts, the brain thinks they are important and that we need to call on them frequently.

Think about what that means to us in our daily lives. Most of us experienced playground taunts—whether literally in our childhood or figuratively as we grew and faced criticism from peers and adults. And because we repeated those "taunts" to ourselves frequently, they sunk in deeply. We used them as an emotional whip with which to beat ourselves. As we got older, we became more sophisticated with our self-taunting. When it came to the core of our emotions, the same illogic prevailed—for instance, we believed that a zit determined our self-worth and that the "cute" boy rejected us because of it. As a result, we do compulsive, self-destructive things because of hidden fears, insecurities, or something some stinky boy said or did to us.

As the years pass, the feelings associated with those early words remain and scratch at our sense of self like a familiar, irritating sweater. This is because the subconscious mind doesn't know the difference between a truth and a lie. It simply believes what we repeatedly tell it. Want a stunning example of how that works? An anorexic looks in the mirror and sees a fat woman. She is clearly not fat in reality, but she sees fat. Believing something about herself actually creates a reality so compelling that a simple belief becomes a life-threatening disease.

We all have faulty ideas about what beauty is—not only in ourselves, but in others. We've formed habits—things we do without even thinking—and they result in the pathways in our brain that convince us we're right. We approach the mirror and instantly zone in on that area we don't like—crooked nose, a zit, a wrinkle, bags under our eyes, a muffin top, a pleasant plumpness, stretch marks. We seldom question if these preprogrammed ways of valuing and defining ourselves are even valid. We just accept them because it's how we are. It's how we've been molded by the methods we've developed to avoid our pain and fears.

Every time we go to the mirror we reinforce the "validity" of what we don't like about ourselves by criticizing ourselves. We criticize our faces. Our bodies. If you do it, don't feel alone. I have worked with thousands of women—from the "perfect" model to the woman who finds her midsection larger than she'd like—and they all surrender to a similar behavior pattern. Would your friends still like you if you said to them some of the things you say to yourself? Really, ladies! Would you even have *any* friends? Numerous studies show the impact of how the subconscious learns and replicates when we criticize ourselves. It's not pretty (pun intended).

So there I was, reeling after my first day of high school in Blanding. I had those habits—those pathways—deeply entrenched in my brain. And what had happened that day at school just proved them all true . . . *again*. I told myself I was ugly and stupid and so overwhelmingly awkward that people couldn't help but laugh at me. And because that's what I told myself day in and day out, I believed it.

After my first day at San Juan High School, I lay in bed, knowing my world was over. Grandma was right. The kids at school were right. I was ugly. I was a loser. I was dumb. I *was* bad. Everyone who had hurt me was right. Who would love a girl like me? I bit my lip, determined to remember what a joke I was—trying to push out any hope in my fifteen-year-old self. I really *was* a joke. I went down the list, being defined by things over which I had no control.

Mom and Dad were horrified that they had accidently given me a whore name. But my mom had a plan for how I could change it all. Her plan, though well intentioned, is a good example of how adults and teenagers don't see problems in the same way. To me, my life was over. To my mom, I simply had to go to school the next day and introduce myself as "Frances" (my middle name). Of course, she reasoned, if I went to school as Frances, all the kids would immediately apologize for mocking me and respectfully call me Frances from then on.

I was right about one thing. Moving to Blanding really did change everything. I knew I would have to go to school the next day—there was no way my parents were going to let me quit and move to the hinterland of Alaska! And then, as I lay there believing all those negative things, something whispered to me, pushing through the spiral of self-hatred.

Not long before that day I had begun to pray—uttering my own thoughts to the God in whom I believed. I believed in *Him*, but I didn't believe He cared for me as an individual. After all, I had proof! Life was hard, it hurt, and people could be cruel! From my perspective now, I can see He was always there—my pain is what had pushed Him out. But back then, I questioned. Something inside was asking me, demanding an answer. What did I mean to Him? What did *I* mean?

So that night after my first day at San Juan High School, I lay there in the darkness and told God everything He had messed up for me. I looked up bitterly. Then an astonishing thought occurred to me. I had to decide what Leta Maughan meant. I had to practice a new way of thinking. This was almost Joan of Arc talk. Maybe I was crazy. *Practice a new way of thinking?*

At that moment, a powerful thought came into my mind: *Everyone in this room loves me.* I hadn't read it in a book. No self-help guru put it there. It came as pure truth, whispered by a loving God. I said it over and over and over again, all alone in my room, speaking it quietly until sleep finally overtook me. A few times during that process I wondered if I was going insane. Could be. . . .

Before I walked into class the next morning, a voice inside reminded me of what I now knew. I said to myself, *Everyone in this room loves me.* How could everyone love me? Suddenly I felt an intense love from my Father. It was so clear: He loved everyone. He loved me completely. And with that, so much was possible.

Everyone in this room loves me. Everyone (breath) in this (breath) room. Loves. Me. I opened the door, and seeing the faces made me smile. They were smiling—at me. With borrowed bravado, I said, "Leta Maughan here!" They laughed, just as they had the day before—but this time it felt like they were laughing *with* me, not *at* me.

It may sound miraculous—and to me it was. That experience transformed how I saw the world—how the world saw me. There was no makeover. There was no wardrobe change. There was no public announcement. There was no dance scene where my awkwardness was whisked away, leaving me suddenly cute. I still had blotchy skin. I still had a missing front tooth and two very large, temporary, gray-streaked teeth. I still had scar tissue. I still wore the same hand-me-downs. I still lived on the corner by the stump. In actuality, though, there *was* a makeover, and it was a significant one: My thought process was made over. Instead of focusing on what was wrong with me, I started to see what was right. Everything was as it had been the day before, but everything had changed because I had changed the thoughts in my own head.

Before that morning, I had made myself the victim because I saw myself as the victim. Life events reinforced how I felt and became who I was. But I was not what I thought. None of us are what we think— we are more than we know. My whole world was different. I could see that now. Eric asked me to be his girlfriend; I let him hold my hand. I was voted the freshman spirit queen. Evidently I could be funny.

You have that same power. If you believe you can walk on fire, you can. (I have; it was awesome!) If you believe you have no self-control, you will eat a pan full of brownies. If you believe you are beautiful, you are. We can think only what we are willing to think. If you open your heart to God and take control of your thoughts, you take control of your life.

Just like so many other things in life, this is easier said than done. We resist learning new things. Change, even good change, is uncomfortable, and even with good intentions we forget to follow through. Those negative habits are ingrained in us. To counteract this, we have to make a very deliberate effort and plan time in our schedules so that our new thoughts will be implemented and have a chance to become part of our brain patterning.

We take the time to reach out to others in loving thoughtful ways. We even pray for them in times of illness or tragedy. But when it comes to ourselves, we tend to be neglectful. We understand that the words we use with others have power—power to help, hurt, build, or destroy. But we seem to ignore that fact when dealing with our own preprogrammed self-criticism. We should be spending time reaching out to ourselves in loving, thoughtful ways, praying for ourselves and our success, as it were, regardless of whether we define prayer as a petition to God or an earnest request or wish.

We can't control the ideas our culture or families will propagate and to which we'll be exposed—but we don't have to buy into them once we know better. In other words, we don't have to live with and accept the ideas that have been holding us back.

Are you ready to let your whole world change? Are you ready to discover what you are really worth? Are you ready to practice a new way of thinking? It is time to banish the boogie men in your life and tap into what makes you awesome!

Hotness Challenge

Do you have flaws? Undoubtedly. Does everyone else have flaws? Absolutely. Flaws aren't the problem. The problem arises when you decide to *focus* on those flaws.

New York Times bestselling author and former Miss Massachusetts, Lisa Kleypas, wrote, "You are your own worst enemy. If you can learn to stop expecting impossible perfection, in yourself and others, you may find the happiness that has always eluded you."

When was the last time you looked in the mirror and focused in on one of your flaws—your crooked teeth, your fat upper arms, your wide-set eyes, or that really big zit? I'm betting it was this morning. Now answer this: When was the last time you looked in the mirror and focused on, even celebrated, the great things about you—your beautiful smile, the light in your eyes, the fact that your hair is the color of a chestnut? I'm betting you can't even *remember* the last time that happened.

If I'm right, you're in serious need of a makeover—a *thought process makeover*. You need to stop being mean to yourself. You need to reach out to yourself in loving, thoughtful ways. You need to treat yourself with the same care and compassion and understanding you use for the others you love. You need to think new thoughts— *especially* about your flaws!

Here's a warning about this first Hotness Challenge: it won't be easy! If you're like me and all the other women I know, you've been conditioned for a very long time to focus on your flaws instead of seeing them in a positive way—or instead of even noticing your really great features! This seven-day Hotness Challenge is going to stretch your mind in a few different directions to get you thinking in a whole new way.

Ready?

1. Grab a piece of paper and something to write with. Make a list from one to five on your paper. Now stand in front of the mirror. Look at yourself—all of you. Look long and hard. Now take a deep breath, and write on your paper the five biggest flaws you notice as you gaze at yourself in the mirror. Got 'em? Yeah, I thought so. Most of us can do that in our sleep. Put the list away for now; you'll come back to it at the end of the week.

2. Each day for the next week, pay attention to the things around you that amplify your insecurities and "inspire" you to focus on your flaws. Notice TV, billboards,

magazines, movies, and other media. Heck, consider overheard conversations. *Really* notice the way they make you feel about yourself. (Not very fun, is it?) Keep a little notebook with you and jot down what you notice.

3. Each day for the next week, pay attention to the compliments you are given. Pay *real* attention. Make a point of remembering each one. When you start this exercise, you might be thinking, *Oh, I don't get that many compliments. In fact, I don't think I get any.* Just wait. Once you're *listening* for them, you'll be surprised what you hear. Jot them down in your little notebook. Each night before you go to bed, read over what you wrote that day. Reflect on those compliments. Accept them. Believe them.

4. On day 7, pull out the list you made on day 1—you know, the list of your top five flaws. Now do two things. Next to each flaw, write a new perspective on that feature—a new way of looking at it, a reason why it's not so devastating, maybe even a new insight that makes you realize it's not a *flaw*. If you need help, look over your list of compliments and your reflections on the things that amplify your insecurities. Second, make a new list: the TEN features that make you an attractive, genuine, pleasant, HOT woman! (Remember: We're not talking just physical characteristics. We're talking the whole package!) When you're done, tape it up on your mirror, your closet door, or somewhere else where you'll see it every day. Remember it, believe it, and live by it!

As you wind up the week, take some time and record your thoughts about your increase in hotness. Keep in mind, too, that this isn't a one-time exercise; as you find yourself creeping back into old thought patterns, repeat the steps until you can once again focus on your positives instead of your flaws. Repeat as often as you need to, and keep practicing!

Chapter Two

THE CLIMB UP
GAINING NEW PERSPECTIVE

Today I am an overly confident, happy, well-adjusted adult, successful in my chosen career, giddily married, and loving my kiddies. But I wasn't at all like that as a young girl. I would not be the chickybabe I am today if I had let the low self-esteem I had then control my life. I am not sorry any of it happened—at least not now, because I love who I am and that I can teach my kiddies through my experiences. Getting to share it with thousands of others is an added perk, and sharing my pain is meant to help you in yours.

There is no way that positive thinking can make everything perfect—yet you *can* retrain yourself to see things in a much more positive way! The difference between the pessimist and the optimist is that one sees the glass half empty and the other sees the glass half full. They both see the glass—the difference is *how* they choose to see it! And how they see it determines how they will approach it.

Remember how I wanted to move to Alaska after that first day at San Juan High School? Well, a year after I graduated from high school, I actually *did* move to Alaska. Why Alaska? I had read a lot of Jack London, and the wild openness of Alaska called to me. I wanted to have my own adventures. I loved the outdoors. I had worked on the North Rim of the Grand Canyon the previous summer, and when it came time to look for my next summer job, I decided nothing could be better than the last frontier. In the midst of finishing finals, I daydreamed about moose, hikes, and the open tundra.

A week before I was to leave for Alaska, someone from the job I had secured there—with a signed contract and everything—told me they weren't going to honor the contract. I needed an Alaska Plan B, and I needed it quickly. Remember: This was in the day before the Internet was a household name. I couldn't just jump on and apply for more jobs. Back then we had things in our houses called phone books. Yes, dinosaurs also roamed the earth. So my mom and I went to the library and looked up the Alaskan phone book on an early version of the World Wide Web. Writing down every contact that looked remotely hopeful, we sent out my résumé. Then I got on that plane! I had fifty dollars to my name.

I got off the plane in Anchorage, still waiting for replies to my résumés. With that measly fifty dollars in my pocket, I called the local pastor of my church and asked if someone in his congregation could use a maid in exchange for a bed to sleep in while I awaited the job offer that I knew would come. After all, I was in Alaska. I knew I would find a job.

I *did* find a family in Anchorage with whom I could stay. And I *did* find a job—out in the middle of nowhere. Literally. It was the only job interview I have ever had where jeans and boots were the way to impress. I would be a waitress, maid, and gas attendant at a two-trailer hotel. There was a beautiful lake and miles of unexplored wilderness—it was pristine! And I had my hiking boots!

But wait. The decision wasn't that easy. The family I had stayed with for the previous week didn't want me to leave. It wasn't just because I could clean a toilet like no one else. They actually liked me and thought I was a good influence on their teenage kids. Standing there in the outreaches of civilization I had a choice: get back in the Subaru and return to Anchorage or stay and accept the job.

I hopped in the Subaru and returned to Anchorage. There were ten boys to every girl in my singles' church group, so my actual job was to date and be dated. But since that job didn't *pay*, I had to find something that did. So I worked at a daycare. It definitely wasn't the dream Alaskan job, but it gave me the chance to have a lot of fun being dated—which was, after all, my primary job. And to my delight, what made me not so hot in Utah—the ability to bench-press 165 pounds—made me a hottie in Alaska.

Dating in Alaska meant a lot of outdoor activities, one of which was mountain climbing. Flattop Mountain stands above Anchorage, and my new friends insisted that I climb it because that was the best way to see the city. I saw no reason not to. I was in shape, and, after all, that is why I moved to Alaska—to explore it.

So one day, we started out on the quest to climb Flattop Mountain. The hill was steep . . . okay, maybe I wasn't in as good a shape as I thought. I had spent the last few months in college, I reasoned—not hiking. Plus I was used to hiking in Arizona's Grand Canyon, I reminded myself—lower altitude, more air. My lungs tight, I realized that Alaska was not like it is depicted on maps. It's not small and off to the side of Hawaii. It is actually at the toppish part of the world, way higher than Arizona and Utah. I was sure everything would be better if I could just breathe!

As the climb continued, it appeared my new friends—who I was now certain were just jerks—were trying to kill me. Perhaps they would leave me here and steal my boots. When did this mountain end and why were they so happy bounding up the trail? Really hating them and my lungs, I found some great rocks on which to rest. I sat down, trying to find the three drops of breathable air available this far above the atmosphere. Small Alaskan children bounded past me with ease and comfort.

As I looked up the trail, I estimated that we were about two-thirds up the mountain. There was no way I could go on.

The people who used to be my friends before bringing me up this mountain saw that I had kicked into self-preservation mode before my lungs burst. They proclaimed that we were almost there—that the top of the mountain was just a few minutes away. My suspicions were confirmed. I could see that "almost" to me and "almost" to them was separated by one-third of the mountain. I wanted no more of their rhetoric: I would be dead, which would ruin the view for me. But they continued telling me that we were almost there and to catch my breath at the top of the mountain.

It was my Jack London moment. That moment where the hero faced the unbeatable, the Alaskan frontier, the wolf, the cold, only to die with their flesh—and, in my case, lungs—eaten by big furry beasts. This was my moment, and I would go out with courage against the odds. I would face Alaska and it would kill me, but at least I would be victorious in my soul!

More realistically, perhaps it was just my pride. Maybe I just needed to show them that I was not a lower-forty-eight wimp (meaning, of course, someone not from Alaska).

I pressed on, girding up my loins for a painful hike. The only reason I kept going was because there were cute boys, but I knew everyone was lying to me. And what do you know? They were right! Less than forty feet up from my near-death experience was the top of the mountain. What I thought I saw from my vantage point on the rock was wrong! The top really was right there. Flattop *is* flat, but while you're climbing it doesn't look flat; in fact, it looks vertical until you reach the top.

My new friends were not trying to kill me after all! They wanted me to see the incredible view—they wanted me to stand at a spot where I could see the city, the ocean, and the amazing landscape that was Alaska. It was suddenly all there before me, but I hadn't believed it. I'd allowed what I could see to determine what I believed. I had to see it for myself.

We believe what we see and we reinforce it by what we think and say. Sitting on those rocks, I believed the optical illusion I saw—that I was only two-thirds of the way up that mountain and that I would die trying to reach the top. Those kinds of "optical illusions" occur in all kinds of settings. Early in my career I worked with brides, consulting them on their makeup and the fit of their dresses. They would stand there looking amazing, with everything just right, but it wasn't enough. The mother and grandmother would tell the bride she was a vision. I would tell her how incredible she looked. And then the bride would hem and haw, finally saying, "I don't know . . . I think I look fat." I can't tell you how often that happened.

One of my first makeup clients was everything society says is perfection. She was absolutely beautiful. But as I worked with her, she deflected any compliment I gave her. Handing her the mirror, I was pleased, thinking she would love the colors and artistry of what I had done.

"What do you think?" I asked.

Looking critically at herself, she said, "I am so awkward; my facial features are all wrong. I am so ugly." I stood there with my mouth open. She was not ugly. She had been a beauty queen, had worked as a model. She had ribbons and plaques to prove she wasn't ugly. But she believed she was ugly, and nothing I or anyone could say would change that.

After she left, I analyzed what I'd done. Had I not done a good job? I'd done everything I could—and I'd done it on a perfect palette!

I finally realized it wasn't my issue to fix—it was hers. I had not failed her by using the wrong makeup colors and applications. The failure—*her* failure—occurred because we worked only on the outside. Her outside was beautiful; it was her *inside* that was being eaten up by self-loathing. She was blind to her outside perfection because she saw only what she believed, and what she believed—that she was ugly—was her reality.

It was then I realized that even the "pretty girls" hurt. The issues I had about me, about what I looked like, about what was wrong with me, were not mine alone. I eventually discovered that *every* woman has those issues—every woman struggles with how she looks!

I never did a makeover the same after that.

From then on I worked on the inside, using the principles I am sharing with you now. I have written this book to share my pain, my story, my inner thoughts, my failures, and my victories, because it is the story of every woman. I believe there is a grand story to what we're all doing here on this planet, and there's great purpose in our finding out why we're here. We are powerful and divine, so He Who Is Stinky (known as Satan in some circles) is trying in every way possible—the media being one—to tear us down, to convince us that we are not enough, to dig a hole in our soul so that we believe we will never be enough. He wants us to believe that even perfection is not enough. Until we are willing to see the truth of who we really are, then we are only climbing, gasping for air right next to the thing that can relieve the pain—a change of view!

One of my childhood friends, Diane Child, said to me, "You can't cover up insecurity." How true! No amount of surgery, makeup, or clothing can change how you feel. Oh, you may experience that momentary thrill. I am very happy when I get a new purse or a new blouse. I like having new things to wear—but that is not the same thing as real happiness. I can feel truly comfortable with myself only if I like myself. And I'm not the only one. Here's the key: *Things* can't make you like yourself. Others cannot make you like yourself. Others cannot validate you enough if you have already decided *you* don't like yourself.

Getting to like yourself requires looking past what's on the outside. Accepting only what you see and never getting past the surface is like looking at a glossy magazine and believing you can actually know a person because you read an article about her. Below the surface—beyond what we look like—is where the real good stuff is. A client told me that she worked to be physically perfect all her life; she maintained her image with diligence. Then, after twenty-plus years of marriage, her husband left her for a younger woman. As I listened, she told me she never let him or anyone else get to know her. She focused totally on her appearance, and that kept others from getting to know her. She spoke with regret when she said, "All that anyone ever thought well of me for was my appearance."

There is, of course, a balance to maintain. We need to look good enough on the outside that the first impression works in our favor—but not put so much time into our appearance that it becomes a burden to us or to others. Perfection is not what makes any of us loved. I love the little imperfect things that only I know about my hubby. Remember, there are those who love you for those same little quirks that make you uniquely you.

It is easy to sit back and wait, thinking life will come to you. Don't. Interesting and engaging people didn't become so by waiting. They went and did. Find out who you are—for yourself. You can do this in several ways. Go to festivals, museums, plays, and anything else that interests you. Don't wait for others to organize it—you start the activity. Take a class. Decide to be inspirational instead of whiney on your social media. Become involved in service and other causes in which you believe. Give your mind interesting things to pursue. If you are interested in what the day holds, you will find that you are a more interesting person, and you will be more interested in other people.

The crossroads happened for me when I began to pray. That was the beginning of me seeing and knowing for myself everything that gives me strength. As a young, insecure girl, wondering if God loved and knew me, I received an answer. It was something that came quietly into my inner being. I believe that each of us is unique and special to our God, the creator of the universe. He cares for the lilies of the field and has counted the hairs on our head. He made it all. He knows it all. He loves it all! That meant He loved me, and it means He loves you.

Discovering our relationship and connectedness to Him is the basis of all truth. As I read from His word, I began to discover truths that science will ponder until the end of time. Those of you who have discovered your connection with the God of the universe know what I am saying. If you have not yet discovered your connection with Him, take the challenge to do so. I don't care if you read the rest of the book, because nothing I can say is of more value than discovering that truth for yourself. God loves you. Pray. Answers from your Father will come.

Put this book down. Go ask your Father if He is there. Until you know that you are a daughter of God, you will never see for yourself the beauty inside you.

Hotness Challenge

In the last Hotness Challenge, you learned to look past your flaws and accept the positives. While that's an extremely valuable exercise, chances are good that you listed only *physical* traits—the things that you and others readily see when looking at you. Here's the reality: What you look like is only *part* of what makes you hot. If your outside appearance is the only thing about you that's beautiful, you're not HOT. Never will be.

Think about people you personally know who are HOT—people you love to be around, people who light up a room when they walk in, people who make you smile. Analyze what makes them that way. They *might* be physically beautiful . . . but they are almost *certainly* interesting, funny, vibrant, and focused on others. And those are qualities that trump physical perfection any day.

In this Hotness Challenge, you're going to put aside physical appearance for a while and take a look at some things you can do to work on the more important thing: what you're like on the *inside*.

Here goes:

1. Make a "bucket list"—the things you most want to do before you "kick the bucket" (in other words, die—hence the name for the list!). Maybe you've already thought about this, but it may be a new concept to you. Don't worry about cost or feasibility; list the things that speak

most to your heart, the things you really, really, *really* want to do in your lifetime. There's no required number: The list can be as long or as short as you want, as long as you include the things dearest to you.

2. Within the next three days, choose one item from your bucket list and plan how you will accomplish it. Be specific. For example, if you want to ride in a hot air balloon, look up the businesses in your area that offer hot air balloon rides. If there are none in your area, find one that's reasonably close. Call and find out the requirements, dates, and hours when rides are offered. Ask about the cost. Figure out how to plan it into your budget. Make reservations. Commit to making a plan in the next three days—then, when the time comes to execute the plan, do it!

3. During the next week, pick a quiet time when you can think and plan. Sit in a comfy chair in a place free of distractions and reflect on things you enjoy and would like to do more of. This isn't the same as your bucket list—these are ongoing things that you would like to do on a regular basis. They're the things that make you more interesting! Maybe you love browsing through museums; perhaps you love concerts; maybe you've always wanted to take a class on anthropology; or maybe you'd like to learn how to knit. Settle on one you'd like to start pursuing right away.

4. Before the week's end, do your research and make a plan! If museums are your thing, find out all the museums that are in a reasonable geographic area. Make a list. Write down dates, hours, prices. Then work out a schedule of

when you'll visit each one—and maybe include the name of a friend or family member you'd like to take along! If you love hikes, find out the best hiking trails in your area and plot out a plan for each. Buy some hiking boots if you need them! If plays or concerts are your ticket, check with local universities, orchestras, or communities to see what's on tap—and follow through with a specific plan. Figure out how tickets can be worked into your budget, and write down the dates when you'll place your orders. You get the drift. The important thing is to *follow through*. Dreaming is nice; follow-through is what makes the difference.

As you wind up the week, take some time and record thoughts about your increase in hotness. Keep in mind, too, that being an interesting, vibrant person is a lifelong process! Once you've done one thing on your bucket list, tackle the next! As you find a new interest you hadn't before considered, repeat the same process to explore it. It's a great big world, and you'll never run out of things to capture your interest as long as you're open to new adventures! There's a bonus in all the work that goes into this process: you'll find that just the *anticipation* of something great makes you a more lively, interesting, and HOT person!

Chapter Three

POOPY TALK OR SMART COMMUNICATION
GETTING RID OF MENTAL WASTE

B Y NOW I hope you realize two fundamental truths: you are a daughter of God, and attitude is everything. Unfortunately, knowing those two truths doesn't always mean we are going to talk to ourselves in a positive uplifting way—but we should!

My hubby insists that *pooperness* is not a real word. But that has never stopped me from using it. One of my motives for writing a book is to see that word in bold, official print because it *should* be a word. *Pooperness*: the act of being truly poopy or stinky; the opposite of true *hotness*. (Yes, I will explain hotness later.)

Maybe you have a difficult time uttering anything that contains the word *poo*. You're not alone. Before becoming a mom I knew that I would be cool—that I would not discuss feeding times, naptimes, or what my child ate. I would still dress nicely and would not have spit-up on me. And I would not, under any circumstances, discuss poo!

Then I had my son.

I love being a mom. To kids, the world is magical. I love seeing them discover something new. The first time my son Nathaniel ate cake—actually, the first time he ate a sweet of any kind—was on his first birthday. His eyes went wide and delight tickled his tongue. He couldn't wait to get another bite. Soon he had created the mess that makes endearing pictures in the memory book. I savor my children. In fact, it's with some difficulty that I am trying holding back from telling you every cute thing they've ever done.

I am particularly fascinated with children's discovery of their bodies. At some point they discover the nose cavity, the bum area, or the front of the bum—and it's then we tell them, over and over, "The things that come out of your body are the things your body doesn't want anymore." As is the case with bodily functions, other things may fall out of us—including verbal, emotional, or mental throw-up, snot, or poo. It is a perfectly natural process for our bodies to eliminate what they don't want. The problem is not that we have waste but what we do with it!

We need to develop mental tissues, mental toilets, and mental trash bins. We let negative thoughts remain unchallenged in our head as though they are valuable simply because they are there. Listen carefully: Not all thoughts are valuable. Not all thoughts are equal. Not all thoughts are going to honor you and your purpose. And not all thoughts will help you be awesome. You can't control every thought that pops into your head, but you can control how long it stays there.

So what should we do with the bad thoughts that pop into our minds? That's where pooperness comes in. The words *poopy, pooperness,* and *stinky* all have a strong meaning. They are words that I can use in a mixed audience of all ages, because we all get it—stinky is bad. Awesome is good. Poopy is bad. Sweetness is good. Stinkiness pops up in our daily life because we live in a human world. So when the stinky thoughts come, what are we to do? Just stand there in shock holding a booger on the end of our finger?

First, we must recognize the power of thoughts and words. Where do they get their power? From us. A metaphor of how this works: One of my son's early wishes was "to have all the powers, even the made-up powers." He loved Spiderman, Superman, and the Hulk. They all had awesome powers. Yet even superheroes struggle with how to harness their powers. We can harness the power of our thoughts and words and focus it on the outcome we want.

How do we use our powers for good to help others? We are powerful beings, but are we using our powers to be awesome or stinky? We create powerful realities just with our thoughts.

A Native American parable that exists in various renditions illustrates the point well. In the parable, a chief has gathered his people and asked them a question.

"There are two wolves inside of me," he said. "One is the wolf of anger, hate, jealousy, fear, and war. The other is the wolf of love, forgiveness, sharing, faith, and peace. Which one will win the battle for my spirit?"

The people discussed the question, debating the power of each wolf. Love was strong, but so was hate. War was powerful, but so was peace. Jealousy was consuming, but so was forgiveness. After much discussion, the people were still unable to decide. At last, they asked the wise chief for the answer.

"The one that will win," the chief said, "is the one that I *feed*!"

It is the same with us. Which thoughts do we feed? I love my hubby. I have also noticed that God made some other attractive men. I notice that—I may even notice for a few extra minutes—but I don't decorate my home with pictures of me with another man. Photoshop makes it possible for me to create a picture of Hugh Jackman looking at me adoringly—but I don't. I could, but that doesn't mean I should. There is great power in saying no. There is great power in knowing I can do something and choosing not to.

I am also aware that God made other attractive women. I am not the most beautiful woman that ever was. I know this, and I assume that Mr. Greene knew when he asked me to dance on August 2, 1997, that I was not the fairest woman in all the land. (In fact, I believe it was my funky-wonky dance moves that won his heart.) He chose me knowing I was human, flawed, and imperfect. Shocking, I know. But that was his choice.

We have the power to choose. God didn't send us down here and then tell us every little thing we needed to do, slapping our hand along the way if we messed up. Instead, He gave us agency. We alone choose our attitudes, our actions, and our habits. You love what you serve. What you choose to feed, what you choose to repeat, and what you choose to do harness your superpowers.

So if you choose to have only good thoughts, are you in the clear? Not exactly. Remember our beauty boogie men? Sometimes bad thoughts surround us even though we choose to not have them. These monsters live inside our minds, waiting to remind us of all the bad things anyone has ever said to us. They often appear when we are tired or frustrated. But don't give up—we *do* have power over them. The thoughts that fill our time are what we feed the boogie men in our minds. If we feed them with kind, loving thoughts, they become less scary; if we gorge them with stinky words of criticism, we may become too frightened to even look in the mirror.

It's important to control these boogie men for more than just our own benefit: the boogie men affect our children as well. Regardless of whether our children are genetically related to us, they are fed on our outlooks and habits. Over a lifetime of being with us, they know how we think. They pick up our ideas about life, beauty, happiness, and money. The story about my grandmother is not unique; others have had people in their lives who should have picked their words with more kindness. My grandmother's was not the only stinky voice I heard—and I realize now that she was speaking out of habit, out of what she'd been fed and thus how she felt about herself. She was projecting what she felt about herself, about her own weaknesses, rather than anything she truly thought about me.

Take on the challenge to control your thoughts as best you can because what you think *will* come out, often like a fart—at the least intended times and at the most embarrassing moments. Make the choice to control the boogie men—those poopy thoughts—and remember that doing so is a little easier than controlling some of the things your body chooses to do!

Hotness Challenge

No one likes garbage. It smells. It takes up space. It's useless. There's a reason they call it *waste.*

That applies to more than just empty egg cartons, junk mail, dirty diapers, carrot peels, old newspapers, refrigerator sludge, and apple cores. It applies to *mental* waste as well—the negative thoughts that bounce around inside your head. Just like dirty diapers, they smell. They take up space. They are useless. Those kinds of thoughts are *waste,* all right. They waste your time. They waste your energy. They waste the effort you could be devoting to yourself and your loved ones.

Time to challenge—and get rid of—your mental waste! You have trash bins and toilets in your house to get rid of the waste that's generated there; time to develop an effective *mental* trash bin so you can clean up the mental waste that might otherwise move you out of house and home, so to speak.

You'll have to do some pretty vivid imagery exercises here, but you're up to it. Ready?

1. Before you can clear out the mental debris that is scattered around your mind, you need to identify it! Sit in a quiet, comfortable place free of distractions, close your eyes, and FOCUS. Focus on what's rattling around in your head.

2. Imagine a trash bin in your head. *Be specific.* What color is it? What does it look like? How big is it? What's it made of? Does it have a lid? Does it have one of those fancy foot pedals? This is *your* trash bin, so it can be whatever kind you want. Just make sure you get a clear picture of it before you move onto the next step.

3. If you're like most women, you've got quite a pile of trash in your head, and it can be overwhelming to tackle it all at once. So start small. For today, locate the piece of trash that gives you the most pain. It can be something you use to beat yourself up (*I'm so fat! Look at that nose—a face only a mother could love!* or *I'd love to apply for that promotion, but I'm too stupid*). You know the kind of stuff I'm talking about. Or it might be something that someone else said—that thing that feels like a knife is being plunged into your heart every time you remember it (and oh, how our minds like to remember those things!). Found it? Imagine yourself picking it up. Imagine yourself holding it in both hands.

4. Now that you're "holding" your piece of mental waste, *get rid of it*! Walk right over to your mental trash bin. Crumple that piece of waste into the tightest little wad imaginable. Now toss it into your mental trash bin! Feel the exhilaration of having it *gone*.

5. Repeat this exercise tomorrow on another piece of mental waste. Keep going, day after day, until the only thing in your mental landscape is that awesome trash bin that has swallowed up all the negative thoughts that were holding you back.

Will those pieces of mental waste ever reappear? Probably. The world is full of ugly little boogie men who like to wreak havoc wherever they go. They'll almost certainly throw some really smelly piece of waste right at you now and then. What you do with that waste will make all the difference—and before long, you'll realize the best secret of all: your mental waste bin is bottomless! It can hold all the waste you crumple up and throw its way . . . and you can move forward, clinging only to the best!

Chapter Four

VANITY PRAYERS
YOUR SECRET WEAPON TO INNER HOTNESS THAT RADIATES

THE EASIEST WAY to get rid of poopy thoughts is to replace them with awesome ones. It might not necessarily be easy to look in the mirror and tell yourself that you are a gorgeous chick with awesome potential. In fact, you might resist doing it. You might say to yourself, *I don't want to get a big head; I don't want to be vain.* I say, be vain! Tell yourself, "I am beautiful."

In fact, I like to spend a little time each day saying Vanity Prayers. What are *Vanity Prayers*? You know those times when you say mean things to yourself—when you're looking in the mirror and staring at your scars, both the external ones as well as the internal ones? Vanity Prayers make those times *work for you*. I'll define them in depth below, but first let me give a little setup.

Most of the time we approach the mirror like it is our judge. But last time I talked to my mirror, it did not respond, "Your Highness, Snow White is the fairest of them all." In fact, my mirror has never said anything other than the words I feed it. It says to me only what I say to it. I guess you could say I have my own enchanted mirror.

You may not realize it, but you have an enchanted mirror too. And that mirror can be used to mold your own spellbinding image. How, you might ask? It happens when you say Vanity Prayers. That's the time you take each day to get rid of what the beauty boogie men say about you and to substitute those false comparisons with the things you know to be true. Don't lose patience with yourself—if you don't know them yet, you will.

Vanity Prayers help you see your own beauty. Even wrinkles—which I like to call *re'dinkles* because it is ridiculous how much we worry about them—can be beautiful with Vanity Prayers.

Let's get into the specifics of how Vanity Prayers work. We'll start with what you've likely already tried, and then we'll expand. You've heard of, or maybe even tried, affirmations or meditating. Picture a woman sitting with her obviously flexible legs unnaturally crossed. She is serene—the very image of Zen. The air around her is soft, peaceful. She can take on the world. Seems great, doesn't it—to be able to have things so calm and clear? If you're able to remove all distractions from your world, great! I can't—entering such a peaceful scene makes my mind sleep or cramp.

Vanity Prayers are for us ladies who live in the real world. I need action, so my mantras/affirmations happen when I'm getting ready for the day—it's multitasking, girls! You're already there brushing your teeth and applying deodorant, so why not maximize your routine? (A man once told me that multitasking was a myth. I patted him kindly on the arm and said, "This lets me know you don't have a uterus.")

But here's where Vanity Prayers really differ from your average positive-thinking session. They require more than just saying random, benign things about yourself. They:

- Require you to turn any perceived weakness or imperfection on its head.

- Demand a new *attitude* in which to do them—one that will change how you see *you*. In other words, that attitude will change your *life*.

Vanity Prayers in Action

There are four steps to using Vanity Prayers:

1. Verbally acknowledging specific strengths, talents, and good qualities you have, just to keep some perspective on how many gifts you can actually claim and how much you have to offer others (this is our more powerful variation on traditional affirmations).

2. Noting the specific things you hate (this is key!), then figuring out—honestly—what is good about them or what they show about your power, worth, and the blessings you've been given.

3. Using the above as a foundation for moving through your day with purpose (pulling out the calendars and your imaginations here).

4. A review-the-day evening routine that honors your honest efforts and puts you in touch with self-kindness so you can slip peacefully into well-deserved rest.

Steps 1 and 2

Steps 1 and 2 are the biggest threats to your comfort zone and may be the most difficult. Check out an example of making emotional and physical scars work for you:

Leta: "I have pretty teeth. I am so glad I had the dentist make them. What a blessing that dentists exist.

"My double chin is my dad's chin, and it reminds me of how hard he worked to take care of his family. It reminds me of the strength, sacrifice, and integrity I inherited from him.

"I am so glad the physical therapist called me 'meaty,' because if I wasn't, he wouldn't be able to work deeply enough into my muscles to keep me out of a wheelchair, and I'd be handicapped the rest of my life." (Just to clarify, I mean this literally due to physical handicaps from so many miscarriages.)

Now you try.

You: "I have pretty eyes. That's a great blessing.

"I am patient (best said with fighting children in the background). I am a good friend. I am a good cook.

"My muffin top is evidence of sacrificing my body for my babies and shows me that I am strong and loving and a good mother.

"My house is a mess because I choose to spend what little free time I have with my loved ones and/or in meaningful activity or development of my talents."

Now that you know what an affirmation is, my suggestion is to replace the time you negate and belittle yourself with time spent being your new best friend. You need to reprogram those pathways in your brain. This won't happen one hour a week in yoga class. You need to consciously, continually, and purposely change your habitual inner dialogue to create a mindset where you see yourself more like your friends do.

That includes all your wrinkles—literal and figurative. (And since you're asking, there *are* ways to get rid of wrinkles. I can name two options right off—you can either pull a Joan Rivers or a Marilyn Monroe. In other words, you can be best friends with your surgeon, or you can die young. Neither of those is that appealing to me.)

Why don't I let wrinkles get me down? Because aging is beautiful. I know that sounds hokey, but it's true—I hope to be a woman whose wrinkles show that I chose to smile more than frown. That's only one example of what I do in my Vanity Prayers—I turn that imperfection on its head. So, when you are brushing your teeth, putting on your makeup, or making sure your slip isn't showing, replace your self-criticism with honest statements about your beauty, value, and power.

Choose to see the good in you, just like you would a friend or daughter. When a friend has a bad day, you look her in the eye and tell her all her great qualities. You encourage her. And if she can improve, you help her see that in a supportive, merciful, patient way. Vanity Prayers will help you be your own loyal best friend—to see your scars in an entirely new and empowering light and to help you learn to change your tone in order to properly correct yourself if you do need to have a heart-to-heart about the changes you need to make.

When we look in the mirror, we reinforce what we feel about beauty and image. I have a friend who often referred to herself as fat and dumpy. Finally, not able to resist, I asked her why she would say that about herself. Not only was it completely negative and mean, I couldn't allow my friend to be treated this way even if *she* was the offending person. Why would she say such a cutting thing to herself? She was tall, with a willowy build. So we had a girlfriend therapy session. (Girlfriend therapy is the best kind. It is typically just the price of lunch, and you know that your secrets are safe. If you don't know that, then you need new girlfriends!) During our "session" she realized that her mother always referred to herself that way—and she believed that what she'd always heard her mother say applied to her, too. We had to see the obvious: My girlfriend was adopted, so they had completely different body types. She *wasn't* her mother.

In my youth I looked in the mirror and saw things about me I wanted to change because of what I heard society say about me. When I improved my thinking, I saw that what was really wrong with me was not what I looked like but how I looked at myself. As I grew in character, I developed a more forgiving heart and learned to laugh—and I got prettier!

I'm glad to be a brunette; despite all the blonde versus brunette jokes, neither is prettier or smarter than the other—we are just different, and that is good. Differences help us see truths about the world we wouldn't have access to from our limited perspectives. Despite these differences, and, in fact, because of them, we all are born with our own unique potential—and we all have access to the same source of truth. We just need to look inside and ask the questions—be they about our value, looks, or potential. We have to stop looking to others, because others can give us only what they give themselves. (In the same way, we can give others only what we give first to ourselves.)

In a similar way, I believe that when others hurt us, they are using the weapon they are most familiar with—the one first or most used on them. If others are critical of you, what are they thinking about themselves? If others shame you, what shame do they hurl around in their own mind? In the end, my grandmother's ideas on beauty and life hurt her more than they hurt me. My grandmother did the best she knew how; her words were just a reflection of what she allowed others to put on her.

When I improved my thinking about myself, I became prettier to myself and others. It is only when we connect with ourselves that we can give our best self to others. When we see the beauty in our own imperfections, we can see the physical and emotional beauty in others and can forgive them of their imperfections.

With Vanity Prayers and the process of change they can bring about, I invite you to look beyond your experience and consider hunting for powerful affirmations that have also changed other women. I invite you to adopt those as things you can tell yourself. Seek out beauty role models—those with inner and outer beauty—who share the knowledge they have gained from that process. One of my favorite poems was written by American humorist, comedian, and journalist Sam Levenson to remind his grandchild what true beauty is. He gave the following time-tested beauty tips: "For attractive lips, speak words of kindness. For lovely eyes, seek out the good in people. For a slim figure, share your food with the hungry. . . . For poise, walk with the knowledge you'll never walk alone. People even more than things have to be restored, renewed, revived, reclaimed, and redeemed. . . . Never throw out anybody."

Let's work on restoring, renewing, and reclaiming ourselves. Use the time while you're getting ready for the day to decide what real beauty is. Start your day by seeking out the good in you. Your makeup is not a have-to; it is a symbol that shows the world the work you've done inside. True beauty is not found in physical perfection but in kindness, love, and in the giving of ourselves—to others as well as to ourselves.

Step 3

Starting your morning with Vanity Prayers helps you start and order your day with the right attitude. Use that attitude when planning your day. Decide on a course of action for the day. Then set your plan in action. Do it with the intent that you didn't just fall into today—you knew it was coming and you are ready to be the woman you were meant to be. Know that you can be the woman that each new day gives you the opportunity to become. Be the queen, the rock star, the chickybabe of your childhood dreams. Be her. Envision yourself doing a great job at the tasks and responsibilities before you.

Starting your day with Vanity Prayers is using the power of your own internal dialog to start your day right. It's kind of like eating healthy food for breakfast. Use it to reform your negative routine of self-punishment, critique, and comparison.

In my Vanity Prayers I also lay my calendar out in front of me (it's on my smartphone). This has a twofold purpose. First, I need to know how to dress for the day. If I'm playing with my kids, jeans and a shirt will work. If I'm going to be doing makeovers all day or giving a speech, then I need to dress the part. The other reason for laying my schedule out is that it lets me see what my "purpose" for that day is. I not only see my schedule, I see the people in my day; I try to put their faces in front of me (if I know what they look like), and then I see me being awesome. I see me being connected, loving, and doing my day fabulously!

If there's an event coming up that makes me nervous or that I have had to prep for, I envision all of my plans going smoothly. I walk mentally through my day, prepping my mind to be amazing. I do not see failure. I do not critique, belittle, or negate myself. I see me doing my best and responding to every situation with my best. If hiccups to my well-laid plans pop in my head, I see myself reacting to them with grace and dignity. A mantra of mine is, "I only have control over how I respond to this."

Here's how it works: after I love my spouse and kiddos out the door, I head with my smartphone in my hand to finish getting ready. Laying it on the counter, I look at my schedule as I massage my skin-care products into my skin. I begin thinking of the clients I will be serving. I see myself being loving and attentive to their needs. I see the sweet faces of my children that I love so much, and I see myself being a great mom to them, connecting to their needs. I see myself as a gorgeous, adoring wife to my hubby, being thoughtful of him and his needs. I go over each face, each event, and see me being how I want to be in that situation. I see me being awesome. I see the day and the possibilities as doable. I will hit the mark of what I expect for me and what those who depend on me need. I have made the conscience decision that as I am getting ready I will do my Vanity Prayers. As I apply deodorant, brush my teeth, cleanse my face, apply moisturizer, and apply foundation, I pump up Leta to be the awesome woman I know she can be.

Step 4

Vanity Prayers are not only used to start the day but to end it. Do the same thing at the end of the day—check in with yourself as you are brushing your teeth, removing your makeup, and cleansing your face. Congratulate yourself and remind yourself that tomorrow is a new day—and that you can choose again to be your best self!

What if things didn't go as planned? In fact, what if they didn't go well at all? Have you ever had a bad day? Despite all your planning, hope, and work, did it turn out to be a stinky, poopy day? Welcome to being human! Because I'm female, I need to verbally process the day's events and feelings. I can get myself pretty worked up at times. (This often happens about the time my husband may want to give me a kiss or two . . . not really going in a good direction, is it?) So my evening Vanity Prayer routine lets me place things where I need to. I ask myself three questions:

1. Have I honored myself?
2. Have I honored those who depend on me?
3. Have I honored my God?

Honor? What does that mean to *honor*? It means you did your best to do what you felt was true. Be honest with yourself. Don't ask if things were perfect; ask if they were honored. By asking it that way, you will see that you did better than the mere events or the simple "to-do list" of the day. It won't always be easy—especially at first—but give it time.

What it all comes down to is the process of becoming. We can choose to look at our life differently and thus love it truly. Here's an example that has inspired me. As a young wife, I was doing the dishes one day. I hated doing dishes (don't tell my kids)—but, really, who *enjoys* cleaning dishes? Grandma Winnie (who wasn't my genetic grandmother, but the grandmother of my heart)—that's who. She loved doing dishes. But she confessed to me that wasn't always the case. She said that she hated doing them at first, but then she did them so much she grew to love them. She was eighty-three when she died and had done dishes for nearly a century. Eighteen years later as I stood in my kitchen, resenting dishes, I could hear Winnie saying in her aged, tender voice, "I just did dishes so much I grew to love them."

Who we choose to become—through how we see ourselves into being—is created by our habits. So often we see success as getting—getting the degree, getting the house, getting the money. I see these things as a side effect of what really makes us amazing. Being amazing is about training your thoughts. Repetition will stick in your mind and help you become the person you tell yourself you are—so do say Vanity Prayers both morning and night!

Hotness Challenge

How you start your day is how you choose to live your life. Begin to challenge the ideas that you have about yourself, about your own beauty, and about your power and worth. Decide to mold new ideas that honor the true reflection of who you are. Create your own enchanted mirror by telling it:

- I am brave.
- I am beautiful.
- I have amazing eyes.
- I love my chin.
- I love my luscious lips, and will use them to be kind.
- I like that I am tall or short. This allows me to stand out in a crowd.

- I am patient.
- I have wild hair like my mom, who is amazing. It's our trademark.
- I am thankful to be a wife, mother, and daughter.
- I am loving.
- I sort of have man arms, but they prove I'm strong, and they hold my babies with ease so I can type with one hand and work on my talents.
- I am a good wife, mother, and daughter.
- I am an example to my children and I will teach them personal strength.
- I choose to do today with integrity.
- I am thankful to be able to learn.
- I am thankful to breathe.
- I like my body. It would be hard to enjoy life without it. Movement is freedom.
- I see the gifts I have been blessed with.
- I will look for reasons to be grateful today.
- I am teaching myself and others through my challenges.
- I see others' struggles and give them love.
- I will speak the truth.
- I crave healthy food.
- I love other people.
- My comfort zone is meant to be stretched.
- I will serve and do new things when inspired.
- I am thankful to be able to walk with strength.
- I am a rock star! (There is room for lots of rock stars!)
- I am powerful.
- I choose today to honor those I meet with a sincere connection.

These are just some of the things you can use for your Vanity Prayers. I encourage you to come up with your own. Now for your two-week Hotness Challenge:

For the first week, say your Vanity Prayers every morning while you are getting ready for the day. If you have a hard time remembering the prayers you chose, post them on your mirror.

When you say each part of your Vanity Prayer, really mean it! Don't laugh or roll your eyes. It may be uncomfortable at first, and it may even make you cry—but as you repeat your prayer, not only will it get easier, but you will begin to *feel* it. Keep practicing until you no longer feel uncomfortable or awkward.

At the week's end, record your thoughts on your increase in hotness. Now move on to part two of the challenge: for the second week, say your Vanity Prayers every morning while you are getting ready for the day *and* say them again every night while you are getting ready for bed. Take some time at the end of the second week to record how much your hotness is improving. Realize that instead of taunting yourself, you are becoming aware of how great you really are.

Chapter Five

WHAT WE SAY WHEN WE DON'T SPEAK A WORD

WHEN WE WERE living in downtown Portland—in a one-bedroom apartment on the fifth floor, just outside of the hip Pearl District—I spent my days discovering the city until my hubby got home from his internship, at which time I headed off to do makeup. I loved living downtown, where I could let my son play at the many parks, visit the farmers market, and had close access to everything.

One day when I was looking particularly cute—you know, good hair day, had on my favorite Capris and sandals—I pushed my stroller full of happy baby and outgoing makeup orders through the line at the post office. As we were waiting, my son threw his cuddly nappy out of his stroller. When I bent over to pick it up, another hand was reaching down to help me. I looked up to see who this do-gooder was, and found myself face-to-face with—Satan!

Sound harsh? Well, let me explain.

He had contacts in his eyes, cheek implants, and horn implants that started at his forehead and continued over the rest of his scalp. Literally every feature of his face had been augmented in some way. And just in case you're not sure of the look he was going for, he had a tri-tipped pitchfork from the top of his ear to the bottom of it.

Being inches from Satan's face was not a scenario I had mentally prepped for. So I fell back on my natural instincts: I started to chat meaninglessly. Thanking him for his help, I asked him what brought him to the post office. Mail . . . oh, good, we were here for the same thing. A lady behind me in the line must have sized up my seemingly comfortable body language and conversational tone, because she looked at me, wide-eyed, shaking her head *NO!* as if I didn't have enough sense to realize to whom I was talking.

He hadn't asked me for my soul, so I made the assumption that though he looked like the mythological Satan, he was not actually him. I'd learned long ago that those who look gruff are often teddy bears, and those who growl are just wounded bears. And those with claws . . . well, they are very grumpy bears. So after a few minutes of making small talk with the character in the post office, I mustered up the courage to ask, "I'm guessing you were not born with, umm, horns?" He'd gotten them in his midtwenties—when, in theory, he was old enough to know what he was doing. I asked how much it cost. I asked if it hurt. I asked how many surgeries it had required. I even asked what he did for a living.

Then I asked the big question about the horns: "May I ask why you got them?" His answer was long and involved—something about God being dead, the universe being the real power, the earth being dead, and people having too many children. When he made that last statement, he glanced at my son, who was smiling up at him, his tongue to the side of his mouth and saliva all over his chin. He was a seriously cute kid.

"So, you don't have kids?" I asked. He said he did not, to which I replied, "That is probably for the best."

He seemed surprised at this response. "Why?" he asked.

And in a moment of spot eloquence, I said, "As far as my son knows, everyone in this room loves him—"

"But they don't!" he interrupted.

"I know that," I said, "but it is my job as a mom to introduce him to the world as he is able to handle it." He looked at me. All I could see in his eyes was a hurt kid that no one had protected. I didn't know what his life was, but I reached out for his arm and said, "I'm sorry no one did that for you." He teared up a bit, but our conversation was interrupted just then by the occasional shift of people in the post office line. He quickly composed himself and put on his tough-guy Satan shell again.

He then told me that people like me were usually uncomfortable around him. "People like me?" I asked.

He smiled and started saying how we were judgmental people—funny, huh? He hurt because we judged him, yet he had chosen to look like many people's deepest fear.

My encounter with that man made me ask what I am doing that prevents others from seeing the real me. Think about it for a minute and you'll know what I mean. If you dress in short skirts and tight shirts with plunging necklines, don't be irritated that men ogle you. If you dress in potato sacks, don't decide that men are shallow for overlooking you. If you pay a surgeon to make you look like Satan, don't get upset if people assume you are mean—or even evil. Remove issues with your image. All we really want is to be understood and loved. Your image, words, and actions can draw others toward you or make them move away from you. Don't let your inner demons rob others of seeing how heavenly you really are.

We have all met people that at first seemed beautiful, handsome, or otherwise attractive. Then, as we got to know them a little more, we were less and less amazed by them. That initial judgment, based largely on physical appearance—what we determine about someone before we have even talked to them—is our "first impression." We maintain we shouldn't be judged by how we look—and as nice as that would be, we will probably have to wait for that ideal until we get to heaven. Reality is, that first impression alone gives us a pretty solid idea about people—how much money they have, how attractive they are, how happy they are, if they are likeable, if they are the devil. It is important that the first impression people have of you works in your favor.

In all my years of teaching people how to dress, I've found it is not the dress that makes the person—but the dress *is* what makes others *see* the person, and then we can go from there to really learn from each other. So think hard about what you want to say to others before you even open your mouth. We subconsciously gather a lot of information about others when we meet them, so how you look, how you present yourself is important—it's how you're seen and judged by the world.

Our appearance isn't the only thing that conveys to others the person we are hiding inside. Our body can speak without saying a single word. Whether we say it or not, we are communicating. Dr. Albert Mehrabian, emeritus professor of psychology at UCLA, says that only 7 percent of what we communicate is actually through words, 38 percent is with our tone of voice, and 55 percent is visual.

I learned much about saying volumes without speaking when I served an American Sign Language mission for The Church of Jesus Christ of Latter-day Saints. The time on my mission was one of the sweetest of my life. And one of the first things I learned was the difference between Deaf (with a capital *D*) and deaf (with a lowercase *d*). Deaf with a capital *D* refers to the culture; deaf with a lowercase *d* refers to someone who does not hear.

The Deaf are not a handicapped group—they are a linguistic group. American Sign Language is a real language, not a collection of gestures. It has all the cultural complexity of any other language. Signs are given for all the words you can find in a dictionary—they're the basics. Classifiers are the spice of the language. You don't merely sign the words for *I drove my motorcycle*; you classify what the terrain was, how fast you were going, and so on. Classifiers give you the feel and motion of the scene described. The third part of sign language is body language, including facial expressions. If your eyebrows are up, that means a question or surprise. You can't ask a question without lifting your eyebrows—that's as bad an offense as using poor grammar. Expression is key!

Why am I going into such detail about sign language? Because the Deaf can teach us hearing people a thing or two about communicating. One of those things is that we need to learn to express ourselves openly and honestly. If you can hear and someone asks "How are you?" you will likely respond with "Fine!" or "Good, thanks, and you?" Those responses are very neat and polite, and no one needs to feel bad or be uncomfortable with messy feelings! It's all very proper, isn't it? But if we hide ourselves behind proper nods of the head and nice little *I'm fines*, we are not only deceiving those around us, we are deceiving ourselves.

Now let's consider the opposite: Ask a Deaf person how he is, and you will find out—he will tell you. When I taught American Sign Language classes, I told my students, "Don't ask if you don't want to know." I made that declaration based on hard experience: As a new missionary, proud to show off my meager signing skills, I asked, "How are you?" The woman I asked answered, describing in depth a recent miscarriage. Trying to be polite, I acted interested for forty-five long, graphic minutes.

People would show up at an event and tell you they had a horrific day. Their statement was often brief, and they often mocked the drama of it. Then they made a sign that meant "move that aside," and they would join what was happening. The message to me was, "Here was my day. I care enough to be real with you, but that is not why I am here. I am putting my crummy day aside. I have vented it. Now we can all hang out together and really connect without emotional fences."

I learned some things about communication that later came in handy. The honesty was very refreshing. I didn't have to try to figure out what someone meant—it was right there in front of me. It was easy to get to know people, their struggles and their joys. It was easier to serve them.

I like being Deaf (culturally). If you ask, I will often tell you how I really am—and just like the Deaf, I can simply say it. I don't expect you to fix it—just laugh with me and be real. When you communicate in this way, you let others know what you feel. You can't keep up the façade forever—you might as well *be* and *become* what you want others to *hear* when they talk to you.

Shouldn't we all be a little more Deaf? You can start right now. Be truthful when you speak. Purposefully use powerful words that are in line with what you feel and what you are communicating. Henry Thoreau said, "Words were meant to conceal thought." When we use words to cover what we really think and feel, we are robbing others of really getting to know us. We will feel lonely in a crowded room because we are not really communicating. When a child comes home from school, a mother knows how the day was by how the child lays the backpack down. It is a sad day when a teenager stomps in the house with a grouchy expression and despondent posture—and, in response to his mother's question, "Do you want to talk about your day?" he says, "No." It's sad because it begins to cut off communication.

Women do this to men all the time. A man asks, "What's wrong?" The woman replies, "Nothing, honey," looking wistfully looking out the window. The man is going to be frustrated. *He asked!* Why do we hint at things instead of answering in a straightforward way? I teach my children that hinting is a form of lying. We have all heard the saying, "Say what you mean and mean what you say." In your communication with others, do they have to read between the lines? If so, you are very likely to be misunderstood—and if your message cannot be communicated kindly, honestly, and in a straightforward way, then you may be the problem.

I had a girlfriend who cried at every birthday and anniversary that her husband didn't get her the gift she wanted or he didn't plan the kind of celebration for which she had hoped. At the time, thinking I was pretty smart, I suggested that she tell him what kind of celebration she wanted and what gift she might like. Great idea, huh? She looked at me as though I didn't know anything—what did I know anyway? I was single; *she* was the married one. "That's not the point!" she cried. "If he loved me, he would know!" She then told me about all the subtle suggestions she'd left for him. The more she talked, the more I was on his side. How was he supposed to read her mind? How is anyone supposed to be able to read our minds?

Some guys are great at gift giving. On our first Christmas, newly engaged, Mr. Greene gave me a candle—a very nice candle—perfume, and a tablecloth. Nothing was wrong with these gifts. He didn't quite know my taste, and his mom absolutely loved the tablecloth. He was buying for the woman with whom he was most familiar. I could spend the rest of my life being sad that the gifts didn't knock my socks off or that they weren't what I really wanted. Or I could just tell him!

Just because *we* know what we want—be it a gift, a service, or a hug—other people, especially men, cannot read our minds. Making them try to figure it out is too much work; besides that, it's just not nice! Don't demand and don't hint. Give your spouse the gift of letting him know what you would like. I give my hubby a list of possible ideas—sometimes I circle an item or two in a catalog—and I let him pick among the options. Sometimes I create an Amazon wish list. And here's one of my favorites: I tell my hubby that my girlfriend Stacey will buy something for me and that he should give her a budget and a check. That way we all win: Stacey gets to go shopping, I'm surprised, and Hubby gets the thrill of seeing me giddy! But none of that will happen if communication does not take place.

Why is this so important? Displaying the wrong kind of communication not only hurts our social relationships but could endanger our work ones as well. When it comes to work, learn how to compartmentalize. I had an employee who was supposed to assist me. She physically came to the office but was emotionally bleeding about what she was feeling. Part of my job is to listen to my clients—I want to help them. I'm kind of like a therapist when I'm helping women through their beauty issues. If I'm guiding them through makeup, skin care, or clothing, I hear it all. It took me a little while to realize that I was paying my assistant to not work! She was baffled:

she couldn't figure out why I was demanding that I wanted her to work at work. In her eyes, I was so cruel! This lead, of course, to me getting another assistant.

What we say we will do is not as important as what we actually do. The desire to "sell" yourself to an employer, a friend, or love interest is tempting, but the other person can almost always see the truth of your words through your actions.

It's not healthy to hide behind false words and actions. Be yourself—you are wonderful! Vanity Prayers are the perfect opportunity to practice tapping into the awesomeness that is in you. In *Return to Love*, American author and spiritual leader Marianne Williamson wrote a thought that is absolutely life changing:

> Our deepest fear is not that we are inadequate. Our deepest fear is that we are powerful beyond measure. It is our light, not our darkness that most frightens us. We ask ourselves, who am I to be brilliant, gorgeous, talented, and fabulous? Actually who are you not to be? You are a child of God. Your playing small does not serve the world. There is nothing enlightened about shrinking so that other people won't feel insecure around you. We are all meant to shine, as children do. We were born to make manifest the glory of God that is within us. It's not just in some of us; it is in everyone. And as we let our own light shine, we unconsciously give other people permission to do the same. As we are liberated from our own fear our presence automatically liberates others. (*Return to Love: Reflections on the Principles of "A Course in Miracles"* [New York: HarperOne, 1996], 190–91)

I think everyone should memorize this quote. I think it should be posted on every mirror in the world. I believed this idea long before I heard these specific words said by anyone. I felt the truth of it whispered to me by my God, whom I call my Father in Heaven.

Love yourself, and others will love you. Dress to succeed, act like you are worth it, treat yourself the way you want others to treat you. If you don't like the messages you are getting back, don't keep projecting the same message. Don't put it out there if you don't want to live with it. Everything in life has consequences; you can't jump off a cliff and complain that gravity has taken hold. If you don't want to splat, don't jump. That is the choice you have. If someone does push you . . . well, try to enjoy the ride.

Hotness Challenge

The first impression you give off is *powerful*—people decide a lot about you based on those first few seconds of exposure, the image you make before you even open your mouth. In that way, physical appearance is important because in those first few seconds, someone will decide whether you're worth getting to know. And if your first impression is favorable, then the fun begins—and people get to know the stuff that *really* makes you HOT.

Like what kind of stuff? Like, among other stuff, the kind of stuff that comes out of your mouth when you open it. Like the kind of stuff you say when the going gets, shall we say, tough. (Because when the going gets tough, the tough can't *always* go shopping!)

This Hotness Challenge calls on you to dig deep and face up to a few of the most difficult communication skills. Your ability to say what you think in a respectful way is one of the most important measures of your hotness—and one of the defining factors of any relationship. In fact, being able to communicate well increases your confidence, relieves stress, and prevents misunderstandings . . . all while upping your hotness factor!

The things you're going to do as part of this challenge might be hard at first. They might make you uncomfortable. Do them anyway. And keep doing them until they're no longer uncomfortable. Then stand back and watch what happens. You'll notice people looking at you in a whole new way—a way that recognizes how truly hot you are becoming!

Ready? Fasten your seat belt, and let's get started!

1. At least three times in the next week, express your feelings openly and honestly. *WHAT?* Yes. Openly and honestly. Even when it's hard. Here's an example: "I'm sure this isn't your intention, but when you check for e-mails on your phone all through dinner I feel as though you'd rather be with someone else." Obviously, you're inviting some dialog. Hang in there, continue to express open and honest feelings with kindness, and encourage the other person through your attitude to do the same.

2. At least three times in the next week, be truthful when you might otherwise be tempted to fudge. You'll be amazed at what opens up as a result. Want an example? "Thanks for the invitation, but I am really uncomfortable going to that particular movie. I *love* spending time with you, though, and I'm totally up for that! Is there something else you might want to do this afternoon?"

3. And here's one of the hardest for us women: At least three times in the next week, step up by acknowledging what you want instead of making others read between the lines! We've all done it. You probably say, "I'm so tired, and this house is such a mess" (hoping against hope that someone will volunteer to clean it), when you *should* say, "I've had a real challenging day at work, and I'm a little overwhelmed by the house right now. Could you please vacuum the living room and hang up the coats while I start dinner? I'd appreciate it so much."

4. At the end of the week, take time to do some reflecting. You're on your way to establishing new habits—new ways of expressing yourself. Record your thoughts about the difference it's making. Write down some of the ways you feel yourself increasing in hotness.

Don't understand how changes in conversation can make you hotter? Just think: The people around you no longer have to tiptoe around, walking on eggshells, trying to figure out what it is you really want or really feel. Instead, they can trust you to be the genuine stuff. And there's nothing much hotter than that!

Chapter Six

―――――――― ✍ ――――――――

HOW TO SHAKE A FUNK
YOUR IMAGE STARTS WITH A PLAN

I F YOU'RE WONDERING how to dress to best express yourself and flatter your figure, we'll get into that in depth in the next couple chapters. But first we have to talk about math for a bit—naturally—because it relates to having a plan, and that's the first key to learning how to manage your look.

So, math puts me in a funk. I don't get it. I have been told that math is a language that transcends culture, time, and alien races. At one point, a friend of mine was explaining that if there were other people on other planets, we could communicate with them using math. I recognized the practicality of the idea, but in my heart I couldn't understand why I would want to establish first contact with another planet using math. They say that a picture is worth a thousand words. Wouldn't it be better to show them art? Some beautiful Monet would set a lovely tone. If things were not going well, we could show them some of our kids' drawings to encourage them not to hurt us. Or maybe we could bake them an apple pie; I think they would respond much better to that than to 3.14 (pi).

Don't get me wrong. I know math is necessary. I love math people. (I really do; I married one!) Math people create amazing things, like calculators, Quicken, straight lines, the pyramids, Excel spreadsheets, and spaceships—which, I just want to say, cause problems with other planets. Have you seen Star Trek? I love things that do math for me, like my husband. I love him. I just don't love math.

I have to use math every day despite my best efforts to avoid it because of early childhood trauma involving multiplication. For me to navigate the world of math, I need help, tools, and a plan. The help often comes from my husband or an assistant who patiently sets up my Excel spreadsheet. The tools to run the business and household finances come from calculators and Quicken. The plan comes from a budget and our goals, discussed and worked out according to our priorities. If you try to run a household or business without the right help, tools, and plan, it's called bankruptcy.

The things that apply in math apply in many other areas. If you find yourself in an image or attitude slump, for example, you probably don't have the right help, tools, and plan. Your image—what others see—is important. You may fight that and say you don't care, but that doesn't change the fact that others will make decisions about your values, intelligence, income, and trustworthiness based on your image. Your image will even determine whether they want to get to know you. You could be pushing people away purposely or unintentionally by the messages you are sending through your dress, hygiene, and body language.

Just like your budget will suffer if you don't have a plan, your image will suffer if you don't have a plan. The first phase of that plan is to determine what conclusion you want others to make about you. Let's be clear here: You do not have total control over that! If someone simply doesn't like you, she is not going to see anything you do in a good light. Don't waste precious time and energy trying to prove her wrong. There is enough success and happiness in the world for everyone, so wish her well and let her live her life.

If you want an example of that, consider me and my family. I didn't have any control over how I was perceived in my family. They exaggerated my failures and minimized my victories. They had a preset idea. There are actually all kinds of examples of this. If someone is a racist, they may not like you based on the color of your skin. If they are terrified of big, burly men (like my father), they will find you frightening, no matter how much of a teddy bear you really are. I remember the time a guy came to pick my sister up for a date, saw my dad working in the yard, and drove off without even getting out of the car. That wasn't my sister's fault—or my dad's, for that matter. Neither of them had control over that guy. What you *do* have control over is your image, and I'm going to share the basic rules of image with you right now!

Image starts with a plan. That takes us back to Vanity Prayers, because they are intended to help you plan—plan not only what you look like, but plan your day. You might look in the mirror and say something like this: *Yes, I knew today was coming. The sun coming up this morning did not surprise me. I am ready to be awesome!*

Vanity Prayers should give you a mindset and a plan for your purpose and attitude for the day. Does that mean that every day will be wonderful? Absolutely not. There will be days when it is too hard to face what faces you. That's why the *prayer* part of the Vanity Prayer is so important. It allows you to give those things that are just too hard over to your God, your higher power, your Father. We have been erroneously taught by the advertising industry that joy comes from achieving perfection—that happiness is for sale. That's simply not true. Happiness in life is not about seeing perfection—it is about seeing perfection in what you have! Those who are happy are those who have decided that what is wrong with their life is not worth being unhappy about.

So, as you plan your day, think about how you will face it, not just what it looks like. You can't control what happens to you, but you can control how long you think about it. While you're planning, plan your attitude. Predecide to be amazing and full of purpose. Happiness doesn't fall in your lap begging you to pick it up. You have to choose it, create it!

Nathaniel Brandon, PhD, said, "The world has rarely treated happiness as a state worthy of serious respect. And yet, if we see someone who, in spite of life's adversities, is happy a good deal of the time, we should recognize that we are looking at a spiritual achievement—and one worth aspiring to" (*Taking Responsibility: Self-Reliance and the Accountable Life* [New York: Fireside/Simon & Schuster, 1997], 10–11).

As you plan your image, remember that it doesn't take a lot of time and resources to look great. It just takes a plan. For example, I have really thick, long hair that takes forever to blow-dry. After children came into our life, my hair needed to be less time-consuming. Now I have a style and cut that looks great, and my hair takes just moments to style. I may not be spending a lot of time on my hair, yet I still present a very professional image.

In the years I've worked with people, they usually assume that looking good requires lots of money and time. There's a reason for that: The magazines aren't teaching us how to make the process easier, they're teaching us to buy things! And look at the models they give us. We are comparing ourselves to people who have teams to help them. I guarantee you Martha Stewart doesn't do it all herself.

I have a team too. They call me *Mom.* Sometimes their "help" means sticky handprints everywhere and no orange juice left in the fridge. Somehow I still manage. But I digress! You will be surprised at how quickly you can fly out the door looking amazing if you simply have the right tools and plan. Your Vanity Prayers will help you get rid of all that negative self-talk and loathing—now you need to get the practical part of your plan organized.

How do you know if you have slipped into apathy about your image? Here's one way to know: You go to the grocery store in sweats and no one seems surprised. We have all had days when we simply have to go get that gallon of milk. I am not embarrassed if someone sees me without makeup—but the fact that they are surprised is a good sign that I am maintaining a good standard on my image.

It's time for you to shake off the funk of your image slump! Get started thinking about your image plan right now. To establish a realistic plan, let's look at what amount of time you are going to spend from shower to out the door. I spend a half hour from shower to out the door—it doesn't take a lot of time or money to look like a million bucks.

Remember, time in front of the mirror is not wasted time because you can use it to do your Vanity Prayers. What *is* wasted time is the time you're standing there, unsure of what to do. Make a list of those wasted minutes. Do you stand in front of a closet full of clothes saying you have nothing to wear? Are you not sure what to do with that eyeliner? Has your hair overtaken your face? Are your clothes not fitting you? Is your skin-care routine not working? In which areas you would like to improve? What areas of your image have put you in a funk?

Did you get a list? That was fast! We are so quick to identify what we don't like. (Clearly you need to work on your Vanity Prayers more!) Time to do something a little more challenging: Identify the *good* things. What are your strengths? What makes you unique? What features would you like to accentuate? Not quite as easy to make the positive list? If you are struggling to come up with some good features, think about the times you are complimented. What have *others* seen in you that is good and positive and strong?

The simple truth is this: What holds us back from fixing our funks is that we don't know how, or when, we need help. We don't have the tools, and we don't plan out what we want. If you want to get started on your plan, listen to what others have to say about you. When others give you a compliment, do you turn the compliment away? Can you accept a compliment for what it is, for its kindness, or do you feel you have to give a compliment back? Others' compliments will help you see your strengths, but that's not all: When you accept the kindness of others, they are more likely to be kind to you again. And every soul on this earth can use some kindness.

Another thing that throws us in a funk is when we assume a particular trait is bad. My father is six foot three and 320 pounds. He is a tough-looking man. As a girl, I didn't want to look like him, but I realized in dismay one day that I had his chin. It's a family trait. We all have it. But that wasn't the worst of it: I had a really big, gnarly scar on mine. Harrison Ford is a perfect example of how a scar is sexy and mysterious on a man—but I'm betting you can't think of a beautiful actress who personifies the allure of a scar. Women aren't remembered in a good way for a scar. You really don't want boys saying, "Wow, dude, what happened!?" I'm often complimented on my eyes, which I inherited from my mom, but never has anyone come up to me and said, "Wow, you have a great chin."

Okay. You've got a good idea of how I felt about my chin. I didn't see my family chin in magazines. It's clearly not my strongest feature. But does that mean it's *bad?* No. I just need to think of it in a different way.

Most women don't like their midsection. We assume it is bad. We don't see midsections like ours in the magazines, and few of us have had people telling us, "Wow, you have a great midsection!" My midsection is covered in an adorable layer of love. That's right: some people call them *love handles* (or, worse yet, *fat*), but I call it *love*. It's the result of my romance with the three Cs: children, cheesecake, and chocolate! Yes, I could change it. I could eat more of the "good" stuff and less of the brownies topped with decadent ice cream. But I don't.

Some women legitimately have a nice midsection because they made a great workout plan and then followed that plan. Good for them! Before you make that kind of plan, remember that some women have a different body type—and no amount of working out will change certain parts of their bodies. If you want to be curvy or you want to be a specific size, be realistic. Determine what is honestly possible. Then evaluate whether you've made a worthy plan—one that takes into account what you can truly change.

When there are things that really *can't* be changed, the best plan of all is to start thinking about those things differently. Let's consider an example. One of my three kids looks like me; the other two look like my hubby. Do I love my children less, or more, for how they look? Absolutely not. I love them because I accept them for who they are. I accepted them for how they came, and I declare each to be perfect.

How do we accept those features that are not our best? What do they symbolize? Let's go back to my midsection—you know, the one that probably shouldn't be bared by a two-piece swimsuit. My midsection has been affected not only by my choice to not love running, but also by many pregnancies. I have had seven miscarriages as well as given birth to the three most adorable children the world has ever seen. (I understand that you feel that yours are more precious, but we can argue about that later.) There is the resultant skin stretching. There is a C-section scar. Those things are there because I chose to be a mother.

Now let's get real about that midsection. It's there in large part because I'm a mother. Being a parent means sacrificing money, sleep, self, and dry-cleaning. It means gray hair and worry lines. It's a guarantee that you will see people you love more than anything else get hurt and make mistakes. You still think an imperfect midsection is the hardest thing? Seriously? I would rather have my kiddos, and even the pain of failed pregnancies, than a perfect stomach. This is the truth—things sag and bag as we age, regardless of whether we produce children. I would rather have the wisdom of maturity than be a perpetual teenager! My midsection's imperfection is a sign of decisions I've made. I chose to not run, and I chose to have kiddos. I don't regret either of those decisions. I don't even regret the chocolate and the cheesecake! It's part of being able to think about things differently.

Once I decided I could look differently at the things I couldn't change, I had such a revelation about things other than my midsection. When I looked at my father's chin, I began to think about my father—the man he is. He has worked his whole life to take care of those he loves. His dream was to be a rancher, but as the youngest boy, he didn't inherit land. He took up another profession, moving mobile homes, to take care of his five kids. He worked in the mud, the snow, and the hot weather. He taught us to work hard, that work has value, and to do our best every day. He taught us that the only wasted effort was work not done right. I was clothed, fed, and housed as a result of his sacrifice, and I am honored to have witnessed the love that was behind that sacrifice. I look at my father's chin now and see that not only have I inherited his facial feature, I also inherited his commitment to work.

I believe in a God who has a plan for me—for each of us. The bumps and bruises of life are teaching me. I don't know everything I need to know yet, and won't for a long time. There are reasons He made me the way He did, and as the common saying goes, "God don't make no junk" (attributed to jazz vocalist Ethel Waters). I believe that. Look for opportunities to thank your Maker for putting you together the way He did. You will find that you will start to feel better when you express gratitude for what you have. If you lost the ability to walk, you wouldn't care as much how your legs were shaped. If you lost the ability to hear, you wouldn't worry how your laugh sounds. When you realize that you can think about things differently, your funk will be replaced with something of greater value. It has been my honor to guide hundreds of women through this process of realizing that what we sometimes don't like in our faces or our bodies can become things for which we have the most gratitude.

Consider what happens when there's a plan. The Great Wall of China was built to demonstrate power. India's Taj Mahal was constructed as a tribute to a favorite wife. The pyramids of Egypt were made to memorialize a pharaoh. Each is unique; each is considered among the greatest treasures of the world. Each has stood the test of time. They all have something else in common too: Each was built with help, tools, a plan, and collaboration between math and art. That's not all: The builders of each of these had a grand vision of what was possible. They wanted to make a statement—be it power, love, or a memorial.

The same can happen in your own life. Be open to a greater vision, a touch of inspiration as you formulate your plan and as you determine the help and tools needed to implement and create the image you want.

Hotness Challenge

Every great image starts with a plan—and it's time for you to start planning! Some plans are for the long term, and they only have to be done once (or a couple of times)—the classes you'll need to take to earn your degree, the trees you want to plant along the back fence to get the maximum amount of shade, the floor plan for the basement remodel. The rest of life? It's pretty fluid—and lots of planning is like bathing: it has to be done every day.

That's the kind of planning you'll focus on in this challenge. So let's get started!

1. By now, you should be getting good at your Vanity Prayers. But did you know they work as an important planning tool? That's right: As you recite your morning Vanity Prayers for the next week, use them to plan your image for each day. Think through what you'll be doing, the challenges with which you'll be faced, and the people you'll meet. Then determine the most appropriate clothing, shoes, and jewelry for your day. If you're going to stop on the way to the store to meet with an important potential client, plan for *that* contingency instead of what you'd usually wear to go grocery shopping. Be prepared!

2. Part of good planning is having the time to do the things you really want (even if that means an extra half hour of

refreshing beauty sleep in the morning!). Here's a case where a little planning now can pay big dividends on a continuing basis: Work on your plan for getting out the door in the morning. Right now, sit down with a small notebook and mentally rehearse your routine. How long does it take you from shower to out the door? Are there places you can save time? Where do you waste time? And what's a possible solution? Let's say you stand in front of a closet stuffed with clothes but can't figure out what to wear. Consider taking five minutes the night before to put together a great outfit. (Don't forget shoes and jewelry!) Does it take you half an hour—or longer—to dry and style your hair? Consider a different, more maintenance-free cut. In your notebook, come up with three ways of doing things differently that will free up some valuable time. Then make a specific plan for implementing all three.

3. Robert Burns famously quipped, "The best-laid plans of mice and men often go astray." In all your planning, realize this: Sometimes plans don't go as planned. Stuff happens. The unexpected rears its head. All of a sudden you're miles from where you intended to be, so to speak, and you're not sure how to get back on course. *That's okay.* It happens to everyone every once in a while. If you plan well, the chances of it happening are reduced, but *it will happen.* So today—and every day—make part of your prayers a petition for help in dealing with the unexpected. None of us has to do it all alone. God is in His heaven, and He's keenly interested in you. Petition His help. Then go forward with your day, full of faith that when you need it, that help will be there.

Chapter Seven

---- ❧ ----

THE FIVE POINTS OF IMAGE
KNOWING AND OWNING WHAT OTHERS NOTICE

So we're agreed your image speaks for you. The effort you put into your appearance has been proven to bring returns. Did you know that women who wear makeup make more money? A simple experiment will prove what I'm saying. Go to the mall with greasy hair and dressed in sweats and tennis shoes and see how others treat you. Go back the next day dressed professionally. You will see a dramatic difference! Why? Because when you project a poor image, others make judgments about you; sometimes they don't even *see* you. On the other hand, a carefully planned and showcased image shows that you care. It shows intent to plan.

My experience has enabled me to boil image down to five powerful points that illustrate the psychology of image. I teach these five points in more detail in my workshops. As you adopt them, you'll see that they are far more powerful than simple helpful tips.

Let's start with a basic list, then I'll elaborate on each.

- **Live with what you say.** Your image speaks for you; do you know what it is saying? What is your personal style? Are you slumpy or sensational?

- **The 80/20 Rule.** Approach your image like a business with a plan and tools, and you will see the success come. Implement your image tools to see your best self.

- **It's not a competition.** Comparing yourself to others is a vicious trap. Avoid the trap! The good looks of others don't take away from yours—there is plenty of happiness and success to go around.

- **Is it too tight?** It's a tragic fact that muffin tops are caused by little fairies that sneak into our closets and shrink our clothes. But wait—another theory is that we refuse to accept the size we really are and squeeze instead into the size we want.

- **The Hotness Challenge.** Are you ready to *be* hotness? Are you ready to stand up to the world and say, "I am hot"? Take the Hotness Challenge and show the world just how on fire you are. (In your case, you will find these throughout the book.)

Live with What You Say

When my husband's military career took us to Lawton, Oklahoma, I got a job selling security systems. It was not my favorite job. But I did it to the best of my ability and soon was the manager. My job was to train and hire new sales people. As you have probably guessed, I encouraged a clean, crisp image for our employees. I considered it to be one of the reasons our sales numbers improved so much over those of the last manager.

Many of my employees were young and didn't *know* what the professional world expected of them. I had a twofold job: to teach skills and to motivate the employees. One of my best salesmen, a young man of twenty, had worked a few jobs in fast food and decided that walking around outside talking to people was vastly better than working a fry thingy. (Guess I just revealed that I haven't worked fast food.) He had a friend he wanted me to hire. I was inclined to hire his friend because my employee was hardworking and teachable, and I figured he wouldn't recommend someone who wasn't.

His friend came to the interview in a sleeveless sweater—the kind you pair with a nice white shirt. However, he wasn't wearing a nice white shirt—in fact, he wore no shirt at all. His little man hairs were poking out. He wore a gold chain and Hanes underwear. I could tell the brand of his underwear because of the way he wore his pants.

There are five reasons people buy security systems: to feel peace of mind and to warn against fire, carbon monoxide poisoning, flood, and, of course, burglary. I explained that to this young man; I also told him that I wanted to hire him. I gave him a little lesson on what a security salesman looked like—someone who would inspire confidence in the customer—and I suggested that he come dressed the next day looking like a security salesman.

He came back the next day. He was on time, yet not a single thing about his clothing had changed. He was wearing the exact same sweater/Hanes combo! I again explained the five reasons people buy security systems and I told him that he looked like the fifth reason people would buy a security system! I didn't hire him. Why? Because grandma would think he was there to case the place—and he was the last person from whom she'd buy a security system. He may have been punctual, but he was not teachable.

When we think of those in a dark alley, we get an image in our mind of what they look like. When we think of a homeless man and a businessman, we get two opposite images. We all make judgments when viewing others—it's in our DNA. We also rely on stereotypes. Think about that—we all have stereotypes that pop into our heads when we think of a biker, a high-fashion model, a construction worker, or a mom. Those stereotypes aren't always accurate—on any given Saturday, a businessman may look like our stereotype of a homeless person. And in reality, many homeless people look very professional. Nonetheless, the stereotypes are there.

There's actually a sort of science behind stereotypes and image. Read any human biology book and you'll learn that as humans we are programmed to first see color, then gender, then size, and then movement. This dates back to when we lived in caves and needed to know what our environment was communicating to us. Red and black = snake. Big black angry bear = danger. We no longer live in caves at the mercy of the environment, but that early programming is still working in us today.

Color

Let's start with color. We all notice color. If you make a value judgment about a person based on the color of his skin, you are a racist. You're not a racist because you *saw* the color, but you are a racist because you used the color to make a judgment about his value. Color is not intrinsically bad—it's how we see contrast in our world. The variety provided by color makes the world more beautiful. But when you wear the wrong color of clothes, the color ceases to be beautiful. Instead, it creates cognitive dissonance—the brain doesn't like it.

How do you know if a color is good for you to wear? It's a good color for you if when you wear it, people say, "Oh, you look lovely!" or "I love that color on you!" When you hold up an item of clothing against your face and it looks good, it is a good color. On the other hand, when you wear a particular blouse and people keep asking if you are feeling well, that's not a good color on you. This is not hard stuff! When you wear the right color, your eyes light up; when you wear the wrong color, your eyes look like those of a sad puppy. Red lipstick may be the trend—but if it's not a good color for you, all people will notice is your lipstick. Wearing the wrong colors will not make the eye flow as it views you—it will make people stare! Now that you're aware of the power of color, pay attention to television and the movies—the wrong color of makeup is often used on the "bad girl" or the controversial character. (See my website, found in the bio at the end of this book, to access more details on determining your right colors.)

Gender

The next thing we notice is gender. Why do we want to know if a person is male or female? Let's go back to the time when we lived in caves—folks back then wanted to determine if they could produce offspring with someone else. Fast-forward to today: you may not be on the prowl for a spouse with whom to make cute babies, but you will still catch yourself wondering when you see someone who is sexually ambiguous. Our minds just want to know!

In the nineties, *Saturday Night Live* had a character named Pat. I *still* don't know if Pat was a man or a woman—if anyone does know for sure, please tell me. The skits featured another comedian trying to figure out from Pat's comments if he/she was a male or female. It was funny because it was so true; Pat's image was so down the middle that we just didn't know. That doesn't just happen on TV. Ever catch yourself looking at someone and wondering, "Is that a man or a woman?" Sometimes you can figure it out without a lot of difficulty. Other times you can tell the original gender of a person even if he or she has taken efforts to change it. But sometimes you just can't tell. Then I remind myself to not look and to not care.

Knowing the biology behind noticing gender can help you craft the image you want to send. In selecting your clothes, the more skin you show, the less authority you carry with you. If you are a businesswoman who is going to present to a room full of men, you will want to dress as an authoritative, respectable woman. A nice, tailored business suit will communicate authority and invite respect. Yes, you have curves; people know they are there. Don't act like you are afraid of them by wearing a boxy suit; just don't squeeze them to the point that anything bulges. No girl power should be hanging out of your blouse. Your jewelry and makeup should be simple and understated, your shoes walkable (2.5-inch heel) but not flat.

Those are the rules for the business world. It's different on a date. If you wear that business suit on a date, you're saying, "I don't really care about impressing you; I would rather be at work." Revealing too much skin says, "I would rather be somewhere else doing more than chatting with you." Completely covering your curves says, "I am uncomfortable in my own skin." Revealing too much says, "I am comfortable only in my skin." You're the one in control. Decide what is appropriate for the occasion, and determine the message you want to relay.

Size

The next thing we notice is size. The language of body size has fostered an industry based on body image issues and weight-loss plans. Size was critically important to the ancient caveman: he wanted to know right away if an approaching bear was one he thought he could kill or one from which he needed to run for his life. Our cave sisters judged a man's muscles to see if he would be a good, consistent provider. He looked at her hips to see how many kiddies he thought she could bear.

The psychology of what makes a woman sexy is in the proportions between her bust, waist, and hips. Have you ever seen a full-figured Polynesian woman dance? Have you watched a slim, curvy dancer? Both are beautiful; the difference is in cultural expectations. The reality is that when determining if one is sexy, the eye of the beholder doesn't care about the size of the hourglass—it just wants to see an hourglass. Think of Marilyn Monroe. She was not a size four; she was a size sixteen!

Movement

Finally, we notice movement. The caveman lurking in the forest waiting to shoot dinner needed to know if the large mass of an animal was coming toward him or away from him. The cavewoman needed to keep the kiddies out of the fire, the snakes in their holes, and bugs off the food. Today, the woman out shaking it up on the dance floor with her girlfriends is more likely to be danced with than the young lady sitting quietly at the side of the room. The beauty of movement showcases, in a respectable way, what God has blessed us with, both in curves and personality.

The 80/20 Rule

Approach your image like a business and you will see the success come! Years ago I was sitting in a sales meeting, and the speaker said the 80/20 rule applies to everything in life. I thought that was a pretty big statement. Really? *Everything?* It's true. And because it's true, it's essential that you understand what it's all about.

The 80/20 rule was born in 1895 when Italian engineer, economist, and political scientist Vilfredo Pareto noticed that 80 percent of the land was owned by 20 percent of the population (see *The Concise Encyclopedia of Economics*). Pareto began seeing this application in everything. Today business coaches, classes, and gurus use the 80/20 rule to hone efficiency. Here's what it means:

Eighty percent of your profit will come from 20 percent of your customers

Eighty percent of your sales will be generated by 20 percent of your staff

Eighty percent of your complaints will come from 20 percent of your customers

Eighty percent of your important discussion will happen in 20 percent of the meeting

If the 80/20 rule really applies to everything—and it does—I decided to figure out some of the ways that it applies outside of business. I know that 20 percent of my dating life led to the courting of my husband. I firmly believe that 20 percent of the drivers on the road cause 80 percent of the accidents. So does it apply to image? Yes: 80 percent of women are not happy with their image and focus on the 20 percent of things they don't like—failing to see the 80 percent that is fabulous.

How do businesses improve their bottom line? They fix the 20 percent. They don't yell at their employees; they build them up and give them incentives for positive production. They recognize that employees will not be perfect but that they can be effective in the marketplace.

Sadly, we often don't behave like professionals. When we stand in front of the mirror, we often give the negative all the power. Instead, let's give ourselves incentives to improve. None of us is perfect—perfection is reserved for heaven, not this life.

Another way the 80/20 rule applies to image is in the way it creates impact. To take your outfit to the next level, but not over the top, 20 percent should be contrasting color, texture, or design. This can be achieved through jewelry, patterns, and, of course, color. Properly placed accessories are a perfect guide for the eye, and clothes are a fabulous way to contour and complement our bodies. (See my blog and workshops for more information on how to pull off this formula.)

It's Not a Competition!

There are areas of life where competition is good, such as sports. Rewarding the Olympian with a gold medal acknowledges that he or she is the best in the world in that sport. But sometimes competition isn't as good—if your goal is to be Miss Universe, for example, you'll have that title for only a year. How many of us are ever crowned Miss Universe? In my experience, four out of five women just want to look good enough to not be made fun of.

Now forget about the Olympics and the beauty pageants and think instead of children's sports. That's a whole different game: each child gets a trophy for participating. It's the same way when it comes to image—we can all be winners. If each of us participates, each of us can win—we can land the trophy and look like the hottie we already are. Everyone wins.

In contrast, everyone loses when we keep score in areas in which we should not be competing. You know who I mean: the overzealous soccer parent who mocks the losing team; the woman who dates Bob simply so Sheila can't have him. When we compete in matters of the heart, broken hearts start stacking up. Love is not a battlefield, and image is not a competition.

Do you go to the mirror and ask, "Mirror, mirror on the wall, who is the fairest in the office?" The evil queen in *Snow White* lost in the end for making her image the pending factor of her self-esteem. She lost her kingdom, her good looks, and wasted a lot of apples. You cheat yourself out on the simple joys of life when you think your value depends on your looks. You hurt others by keeping them from really seeing your value—but, even worse, you fail to see the areas in which you should be competing, like your personal character. Pushing yourself to be the best you can be in your values and morals always reveals your true worth. That's an area in which we all win. We can all be champions. As just one example, we can all be honest; no one loses when we are true of character.

Think about why you are loved. Why do your parents love you? Do they love you because you are the most beautiful student in your school? Or do they love you because they chose to comfort your cries and feed and clothe you for eighteen years? Did your spouse marry you because you are Miss Universe, or did he pick you from among all others because of how you made him feel when he was with you?

Each of us is unique. We have our own body type, coloring, facial structure, and personality. Of all the billions of people on earth, no two of us is exactly the same. With billions from which to choose, who can say which of all those variations is the best? Even in the world of fashion, no one can decide: fashion changes every six months! You are the best you, as Dr. Seuss says, "Today you are youer, that is truer than true. There is no one alive who is youer than you!" (*Happy Birthday to You!* [New York: Random House Books for Young Readers, 1959]).

One of my mantras goes like this: "There is enough success and happiness for everyone!" As women, we dress to impress other women. Remember, we are not competing with other women. Ladies, let's give each other the permission to be our own unique kind of beauty. Let's celebrate the traits that make us all beautiful in our own way.

You know those people, the ones we compare ourselves to—the ones with the perfect lives? You know her: the mom down the street whose children seem to always say please and thank you, whose children dress in color-coordinated outfits with bows and socks that match, who is perfectly trim. How does she do it? You know her, too: the girl who gets perfect scores in school. Well, consider this: perhaps the lady with the manicured children wakes up earlier than all the rest of us so she can get everyone (including herself) all fixed up. Maybe the girl with the perfect scores studied harder, or maybe she's just smarter in a particular area. Life is not fair. We have a tendency to compare the worst in us to the best in others. It's the ultimate of an unfair comparison.

Because life isn't fair, we all have different skills, interests, and talents. It's not unfair that some do better at one thing when we all have our own thing we are good at. As a kid I couldn't see my talents because they didn't fit on a stage. I couldn't play an instrument and was too shy to do what I really wanted—to be in a play. I actually did perform in a play once—I was in the background with no speaking parts. There was Lily out front, singing the part; she was beautiful, talented, and smart. I thought she was really nice. And she was. She had also practiced her talent and had earned her spot.

So get rid of the sense of competition—and the jealousy that comes along with it. Jealousy only prevents us from learning about and from each other. Instead of being jealous, shine at those things you alone are good at.

Is It Too Tight?

Magic fairies *do* exist; I *have* been to Disneyland. But even fairies can't change the size we are.

It's a common scenario: We lay on our beds trying to force the jeans up, suck our stomachs in so we can button the jeans, and spend all day in pain because they are so tight. At some point during the day, we see our reflection and are shocked to see a muffin top. *That's it!* we tell ourselves. *I am fat!*

Enough with the poopy image talk! You would be perfectly lovely if you bought jeans that fit you properly. How do you know which pants fit properly? I suggest choosing pants that fit on the top of your hip bone, as bones do not change through a monthly cycle of water retention and hormones. That's not all: they are also much more comfortable than pants that squeeze the soft midsection where your intestines, stomach, liver, and other guts reside.

We get so attached to a specific size—usually the size we once were or the size we want to be. Remember that size labels vary according to manufacturer and brand. What cultural ideas have given us a perception that we are supposed to look a certain way in order to attract the right husband? That is just as damaging as the culture in China that determined a certain size foot was beautiful—and, as a result, promoted foot-binding!

Certain ideas can strangle us, bind us in mental ropes of false perception, prevent our lungs from getting the needed air, and rob us of hope at the lack of oxygen. Be willing to cut the ropes that hold you back from improving your ability to breathe. Success in any venture comes to the person who believes that she can achieve it and then works to obtain the prize like she would fight for air.

When it comes to clothes and how we see our image, we can do more when we think we can. Common objections are: *It takes too much time and money. I don't really care. It's just the way I am. It's other peoples' problem—they are just too judgmental!* No one can make us feel a certain way. I hope to motivate you to improve your image, but true image is only improved when the inside is worked on too. If you don't feel beautiful, you won't see beauty when you look in the mirror. If you see yourself as a bad person, no kind words or compliments will make you feel better about yourself. You need to question the ideas that are constricting you.

We will all have struggles, heartache, and pain in life. The trick of life is to not be the cause of our problems. Problems will find you—but where you place your focus and energy will help minimize the effect of those problems and will help you see your way through them. You hold the ropes of your life—don't let them hold you. Where you focus, what you choose to see, and what you think about will become the course of your life. As you look ahead, you will see one of two things—either a bright horizon or an endless expanse of dirt. It all depends on where you look. Will you look up or down? It's your choice!

True Hotness Defined

Change in any form is scary, uncomfortable, and, depending on your personality, to be avoided. I want you to implement the things you have learned in your daily life—and if no change occurs, you have wasted your time and money. Whatever your motivations for seeking out this information, only you can choose to learn and do—unless of course you hire a beauty team, a makeup artist, a stylist, a personal chef, and a personal trainer. My beauty team comes in my bathroom every morning and steals my hairbrush, takes my favorite shimmer eye shadow, and uses the shower just when I plan to. They also call me mom and wife. What better motivation could you have for giving others your best image?

I am known as "Hotness." There are two kinds of hotness. There's the kind of hotness that because of its heat and lack of control burns everything it touches, leaving destruction in its path. It sizzles and teases and leaves those who touch it burned, scarred, or dead. As mesmerizing as the patterns it weaves are, it's still a hot mess out of control. No one wants to be that kind of hotness.

The other kind of hotness is heat that is kept in control. It can be lifesaving to a weary traveler. It warms food and provides safety. It draws others to it because of the warmth it gives off and the security it provides. Nothing feels better in the coldness of life than to be warmed with the heat of hotness that knows how to give and serve those close to it. That's my kind of hotness.

Fire in its designated place can be the difference between life and death. Fire out of control destroys everything in its path, cutting down the beauty of its environment. Using our hotness correctly will attract others to us to enjoy warmth and conversation.

One day, at a workshop I was about to teach on the psychology of beauty, a woman seemed surprised that I was the presenter. She said, "I thought you would be thinner and prettier." I laughed; I thought that was hilarious. The other women hearing this seemed confused at my reaction to such an insensitive comment. I actually love that she said this—she thought only perfect women could teach about beauty. It gave me the opportunity to change her perception. After my speech, she thanked me and complimented me on my hotness. She had learned that we are all hotties. I want you to give yourself permission to see your own style of hotness and to let others possess their own hotness too!

When we embrace our own hotness, it not only makes us feel good about ourselves, but it helps others too. We have talked about the power of the words we say to ourselves during our Vanity Prayers. The Hotness Challenge is to go out and give that power to others! According to renowned psychologist Dr. John Gottman, known for his work on relationship stability, we need to hear five positives for every negative we hear. How we speak to others not only reveals our own inner dialogue but can influence theirs. Can you remember a compliment from a respected teacher? The words hang around us; we remember them. Becoming a person with a *habit* of positive language comes from positive thinking.

Transitioning from the negative will take practice! Never diminish your own hotness! Or that of others!

When someone asks how you are, instead of saying "Fine," steal my response of "Fabulous!" or "Insanely great!" It will make others smile, giving you the attractive quality of being a positive person, which will in turn make you feel even more fabulous! I use overly-positive language when referring to my husband and children. My terms of endearment for my husband are Sexy and Lover, and I refer to my children as Awesome, Prince, Hero, Princess, and Sweet One. One day as I was directing my children in a task, my son stopped what he was doing and said, "Which Awesome?" Isn't that a great thing to be confused about? To which one of us awesome and amazing children are you referring? If you have children in your life, remember their tender self-esteem is still being molded. Take great care with how you treat them.

As adults, our self-esteem is our responsibility. Don't be so quick to give up your power to others by letting their stinky, poopy words have any effect on you. Throw out the things that leave you feeling powerless, empty, and hurt. And whatever you do, don't throw out negative thoughts to others; if you do, you are telling them you don't want them in your life. How we communicate will dictate the quality of our relationships. How do I refer to my friends and others? When I pick up the phone and see that it is my friend, I say, "Hey, Hotness!" I have never had a friend or client offended by my cheesy kindness. In fact, it is irresistible!

Hotness is my word. I like how it sounds, how it rolls off the tongue, and how it makes me feel when I say it. Mostly, I love how others smile when they hear it. I didn't choose the word *hotness* by mistake. Have you ever stared into a fire? The intensity and vibrancy of the flame is mesmerizing. It's so delicious to curl up near a fire and feel its warmth. Friends and family are drawn to linger; soon marshmallows are toasting, and conversation is flowing.

We cannot force our hotness on others; they either want the heat or they don't. Some just want to stand in the cold and freeze; if we force our warmth on them, we will burn them. Each gets to choose how close he or she wants to stand near sources of heat. Only those who are willing and prepared for the hotness—often those closest to us—can share in the spark of what we know. Fire can be shared, and when it finds a receptive source, it grows. Like love, it is never weakened by being shared. It only gets stronger.

Almost anything can burn, depending on the heat source and the accelerant used. Hotness can become the ultimate source of power for good and bad. Throwing our hotness around indiscriminately will cast dangerous sparks into our environment that could turn on us and leave us burned. Your hotness, your good looks, are not a plaything with which to tease others. Use your hotness wisely, and you can light up a room by just walking in.

Will you take the Hotness Challenge? Look for your own unique ways to share your vibrant flame of hotness. When you get good and can stoke the flames of your own hotness, you become mesmerizing and will attract others to want to share your spark! There is no greater feeling than knowing you helped another's hotness grow—that because you shared, that person now possesses something that will warm him or her during the most chilling winds of their own life path. Be a good friend to yourself, be a good friend to all who are blessed to be near you, and be surrounded by really great, amazing, loving, and fabulous people. I welcome you to create your own flame of awesome hotness in your life!

Hotness Challenge

If you read this chapter carefully, you know about the 80/20 rule, and you know an important way it applies to us as women: far too often, we focus 80 percent of our attention on the 20 percent of things we *don't* like about ourselves—and, in the process, we fail to see the 80 percent of things about ourselves that are flat-out fabulous.

In other words, we give the negative all the power.

We expend an astronomical amount of time, energy, and effort on the handful of things about ourselves that, in the long run, don't matter. Why don't they matter? No one can achieve perfection. It's simply not possible. (We could really argue that it's not even *desirable*.) If the percentages hold up—and they *do*—there are four really terrific things about you for every one thing that's maybe not the best.

Want a real-life example of a better way to approach life? Watch a two-year-old. So what if the clothes don't match? Who cares if the hair's a mess? So what if the teeth—the ones that are even there, for crying out loud—look like a staggered row of crooked pegs? Chances are good that you'll see real joy! She'll dance for all she's worth, regardless of who's looking.

In this challenge, you're not going to fix the 20 percent. That's not the point. You're going to switch things up by focusing on the 80 percent of things about you that are flat-out fabulous. And hear this very clearly: I'm not just talking physical attributes, like skin and teeth and eyes and hair and weight. Those things figure in, of course, but they're trumped by other things that are much more important: your character and your values.

So here goes:

1. Let's start by getting the worst part over with. Make a list of the things you don't like about yourself. It should go pretty quickly—most of us are pretty adept at that. Now stand up, rip your list into a bunch of little pieces, and throw it in the garbage. Throw out the things that make you feel unattractive, powerless, hurt, or empty. You're *none of those things.*

2. Now make a list of the things about you—the estimated 80 percent!—that are flat-out fabulous. You have them, you know. We all do. I'm guessing this list won't be quite as easy to write because chances are good that you've spent a *lot* of time ignoring the things about you that are good. But keep at it. If you get stumped, ask your loved ones to help. They know a *lot* about what makes you the wonderful person you are.

3. By now you've been practicing Vanity Prayers. You're probably getting pretty good at them. Well, now you have some new fodder for those Vanity Prayers: your good qualities! You're going to use those things in your Vanity Prayers from now on. Starting tonight, choose one thing from your list. It could be the color of your hair or your ability to make others smile or how well you play the piano. Whatever you choose, add it to your Vanity Prayers. Celebrate it. Keep it at the top of your list morning and night for two days.

4. On the third day, choose another good quality from your 80 percent list. Add it to your Vanity Prayers. Celebrate it. Keep it at the top of your list morning and night for two more days.

5. Keep going.

You get the idea. Rotate through that 80 percent list—the qualities that make you *hot*! And you'll notice an amazing thing: you'll start feeling hotter than ever. Reflect on that. Jot down your feelings about your increasing hotness. And keep it up! Become a trendsetter and see what's right with you instead of what's wrong. Be positive in a negative world!

Chapter Eight

---- ❧ ----

PUTTING TOGETHER YOUR LOOK
BEAUTY SECRETS OF THE PROS

CLOTHES SPEAK FOR YOU. Dressing well and selecting appropriate clothing shows professionalism and planning. No one wants to end up looking like a badly stuffed sausage! Benjamin Franklin said, "If you fail to plan, you are planning to fail." We are not sure how much Mr. Franklin knew about style, but we can all agree that the most efficient and least painful way to find items that make you squeal is to have a plan. Here are my organizing and shopping tips to help you get going on your plan.

Start with what you have. Contentment is a part of finding happiness. If you are only willing to put effort into your appearance when you are a certain size, or if you are a procrastinator, stop now— you are worth your happiness today. And those who love you want you to be happy and embrace your hotness.

Closet Overhaul

I love clothes. I admit that it is a genetic (hoarding) trait that runs in my family. The first time I had a client with only ten things in her closet, a part of me cried for her. She *literally* had nothing to wear. If your closet is overflowing with items, you have a different problem: You have something to wear—you just can't find it.

To organize your closet, grab a girlfriend and help each other out. First, without judgment, critique, or any poopiness, organize your clothes following these steps:

1) Season
2) Purpose
3) Color
4) Fit
5) Happiness factor

Start by taking everything out of your closet—everything! This is so you can really vacuum and dust—plus, you may find that missing sock in the crevices. It will also give you access if you need to add a shelf or hanging extension.

If your closet is small, you need to be creative in your system— use your space wisely. Utilize backs of doors, floor space, and all interior walls. Go to Ikea or a closet organizing store on or offline. Hang shoe racks on the back of your closet door. Door hangers with multiple hooks are also a good solution for hanging bathrobes, belts, hats, and scarves. It's possible that no matter how much you try to organize, you may simply have too much stuff to fit in your closet. If you have a walk-in closet and you can't walk into it, you have too many clothes. If you have a very small closet, you will need to rotate your clothes by season.

Now that everything from your closet is on your bed, get rid of the things that don't fit, that you don't like, or that you simply no longer want. Then you'll need to put the rest of the stuff back in your closet. Things should be put back into your closet in this order:

Season

Hang short-sleeve shirts in prime closet location since they can be worn all year long paired with sweaters and blazers and layered with longer sleeves. Place heavy-weight clothing items with their wintry friends that can be shifted quickly as the weather changes.

For example, in my closet I start with my summer pants and short-sleeve shirts. Next to those are my skirts, dresses, sweaters (hung properly), blazers, and coordinated pieces. Below the summer pants are the fall and winter heavier-weight pants and my long-sleeve shirts.

Purpose

Pairing your items properly completes a put-together look. Blazers do not go with T-shirts. Grouping your clothes by type will help you get dressed quickly and appropriately for the purpose of the day or event. Some examples of "purposes" would be clothing for business, date night, parties, or exercise. The dingy stuff you paint in doesn't belong in your closet to tempt you when you have the flu—it belongs with the painting supplies.

When my children were little, the dry-cleaning items were not used as often—it was a phase of my life—but I still got dressed up for work. I left clothes that needed to be dry-cleaned in my closet, but I put a scarf over them so no dust accumulated on the fold or the shoulders. As my children grew, these items moved forward into the prime location that previously held jeans and casual blouses.

Dressing to the purpose of the day is a symbol of being ready. It is better to be overdressed, to an extent, than underdressed. Just as our body language shows off our confidence, so does our style. As you assemble your outfits, be aware of how you put things together. What you wear demonstrates your values and communicates what you will and won't accept. Lastly, make sure your outfit is appropriate for the occasion. If you are going to a wedding, dress up. If you are going to a funeral, don't wear red.

Taking proper care of your clothes will help them serve you longer. Don't assume that you know how to take care of a piece of clothing—read the label carefully, preferably before you buy it.

Color

What goes with what? You can quickly see what your options are when colors are grouped together. Group your clothing in each purpose category by color—blacks, browns, mustards, purples, reds, greens, and so on. Using the right colors will enhance your skin and hair and will make your eye color pop!

You don't need twenty-one flavors of color in your closet. I have what I call *core colors*. They are the colors you build around: black, brown, and navy. You may only have two of these colors, or you may have all three. The basic classic pieces should be in the core colors. I call the other colors *key colors* because they turn it all on. I love black; it shows off makeup. But I don't want to be in all black every day—people may confuse me for a ninja! Pair a black suit with a pop of color, a mix of texture, or a complimenting pattern for a style that will stand out—in a good way.

You only need three to five key colors. That's it—if you want more, that's okay. Just start with having the accessories, purse, shoes, and jewelry that are either in your core color or in the best key colors for you.

Fit

If it doesn't fit you right now—today—it has no place in your closet. Let me repeat: if it doesn't fit you, it doesn't belong in your closet. In your childbearing years, you have two years to get back into your previous size of clothing. If you're not there after two years, don't look at every item, mourning your prior size. Swoop them up and bless another woman's life with a new wardrobe. Send them to a neighbor, friend, women's shelter, or the Goodwill. (If you get in even better shape later, then you get to go shopping. How exciting is that?)

As you put things back in your closet, try on each item. This is the *most important* step! Make sure it still fits well, with no strained fabric pulls, tears, beading, discoloration, pitting, or loose threads. If it's too tight or just plain outdated, get rid of it! Instead of hanging on to your "skinny jeans" until you lose a few pounds, donate them. Then, when you get down to your goal weight, treat yourself to a new, stylish pair of jeans. If the item is in good condition and still fashionable, think about selling it at a local consignment store. I like to just give my clothing that no longer fits to a friend. Who doesn't love a new-to-them freebie? Once I was able to give a whole wardrobe to a young lady who was entering the workforce. That made parting with my old friends feel gratifying.

When someone looks at us, they see the shape, not the size. When I was pregnant, I didn't want people to know, as I often miscarried, so I hid my pregnancy under clothes. Prechildren, I was a size eight or ten. As I grew in my pregnancies, I moved out of that size to twelve, fourteen, sixteen, and then finally into maternity clothes. I looked great—and because I worked as an image consultant, makeup artist, and presenter, others were "checking out" my image and presentation more than most. I had to look good, and I didn't want to talk about how far along my pregnancy was.

Once, a group of teen girls was telling me how skinny I was and how cool that was. They couldn't have known that I was three months pregnant. No little bump gave me away. Dressed differently it would have been obvious, but I used the clothes as a tool. As I moved up in size I took the clothes that no longer fit out of my closet and put them in plastic bins labeled by size. Only what fit hung out in my closet.

Happiness Factor

If it doesn't make you happy, if you don't feel fabulous in it, why keep it around to mock and torment you when are trying to get ready for the day? Why risk wearing something that really just makes you sad? You have a pile of items that you know are not for you; donate them or give them away. I recommend letting your girlfriend decide which pieces of clothing should go, as you may get too wrapped up in the emotion of a particular piece.

The day my hubby proposed, we took a picture. I was wearing a flowy shirt that was trendy at the time, and I looked very cute, but I didn't love it. For some reason, that shirt hung in my closet far too long. Too bad I didn't donate it to a playhouse for a romantic play. Sentimental value doesn't need to reside in your closet; it lives in your memory book and your heart. (Sniff . . . feeling the love?)

If you have not worn a piece of clothing for a year, then it is not speaking to you—unless, of course, it is saying, "I make you feel frumpy." Or it may not feel like you, even though you *want* it to be you. It has spent its whole life with you being put on, being taken off, and never being seen outside your bedroom.

Now your closet is clean, the bad clothes are gone, and the rest are waiting for some new companions—items that will make you even more fabulous than you already are. It's time to go shopping. But wait! Don't just run to the mall and pull out the plastic. You need to be in control when you are shopping. I have a great way I do this. I call it the Power Notebook.

The Power Notebook

My Power Notebook used to fit in my wallet along with paint chips of my colors (the ones that look good on me); now it's all on my smartphone. Regardless of what format you decide on, a Power Notebook contains:

- *Your colors.* Only buy what is hotness for you! Knowing the colors you look great in is an artistic thing. If you are more of the math type, art may be a little confusing for you. If so, ask your friends which colors look best on you. (I also teach workshops on the tricks for finding your best colors, and you can find more in-depth information on all the topics in this chapter on my blog.) Notice what people compliment you on. The right color is important.

- *The things you need.* Do you need a pair of black slacks, a camel blouse, a red sweater? Have a shopping list ready that you compiled during all your closet organizing.

- *What you are willing to spend.* Core (classic) pieces are worth spending more on than trendy items.

- *Style ideas.* I collect pictures on my smartphone of looks I want. Spread the love by asking women whose look you love if you can take their pictures. It will make their day, and they usually know where they got it and how much it cost.

Now when you walk in the store, instead of acting like you have no idea what you are doing there and avoiding the sales clerk like she is contagious when she chirps, "How may I help you?" your answer can be, "I am looking for this color, for this much, and in this style. Do you have it?" The sales clerk already knows what is in the store! If that store doesn't have what you're looking for, go to the next store. You're not only organized, but you are also efficient!

Your Power Notebook gives you a plan—and having a plan will help you save money. Shop sales with specific items and colors in mind so that you don't buy on impulse; stick to your plan. Don't turn up your nose at secondhand options. And remember the most important rule: Buy only what fits you right now!

Makeup

In addition to clothing, there are other items you need to consider when putting together a look that is all you. Makeup is a great tool but should be used so that others can see you, not the makeup. Have you ever seen someone and wondered if they were pretty or just really good at makeup? If you put on too much makeup, all others will see is the buildup and flashy colors. Makeup should draw people into looking into your eyes, which is where your true hotness is. Allow others to see your best features. If your makeup is enhancing, you will look like you have it all together in something as simple as jeans and a blouse.

Classic makeup application allows *you* to be the focus, not the makeup. There are two kinds of makeup artists: those who show their skill, and those who show off you! Learning to put on great everyday makeup properly is simple. As makeup artists, we work on the most beautiful canvas that God has made, and an infinite number of different combinations makes each of us completely unique. It is never boring to find that right balance between structure, coloring, and a woman's own personality to enhance and emphasize what will show her own hotness!

During my blue-collar childhood, I didn't even know that makeup artists existed. I knew that I was clueless about makeup, and my mother's limited use was no help—she used her lipstick as a blush. A quick smudge of color on her cheeks and a smack of her lips and she was done. With a scar through the right side of my lip, a large one straddling my chin bone, and a bump on my forehead that took years to even out, I had slightly higher hopes and needs. A little bit of lipstick wasn't going to cut it. Also, I was plagued with dry skin and sensitivity to most products we had at home. Later I learned I was sensitive to most things in the marketplace.

Wearing flannel and blue jeans, sitting at my first makeup counter, I felt completely out of my element. No one else was wearing flannel and blue jeans. I was regarded with pursed lips as an array of products was layered on my face. Having never applied anything to my eyes, the unfamiliar sensation of brushes and liner caused blinking, twitching, and tears. When the artist was done telling me the latest and greatest that I needed for my sixteen-year-old face, I looked in the mirror, ready for success as a—streetwalker?! She may have done a good job, but it was way too much for me. I needed more of a skin-care lesson and less color intensity.

I have never forgotten what it feels like to be humiliated by my makeup and at the same time captivated by the potential. The scar on my lip was unnoticeable under lipstick, and the funkiness on my forehead disappeared under foundation—but I could SEE the lipstick and the foundation. Which was worse? Seeing so much makeup or seeing the scars and skin issues? There are no pictures to document this first look. I washed it all off in the mall bathroom. I went with a boy to the dance wearing bold brown eye shadow and a slightly pigmented lip gloss from the drugstore. Bold and crazy, I know. And no, I wasn't wearing flannel; I borrowed my mother's dress. Yes, I was a trendsetter.

My mother taught me that if I didn't know something to ask questions, do research, and read about it, so I did. My fascination with makeup was something I did more on others than myself because I soon started getting little puffy sores around my eyes. If I didn't wear makeup often, it didn't irritate. But what I couldn't tolerate, others could—and I was enthralled with putting these amazing paints on other people. It was a lot of fun!

At the time, my makeup goals were simple. Number one, not be made fun of. Number two, look cute. And number three, someday have a boy kiss me. Entering college, I'd accomplished number three. I was struggling with consistency on number two as my skin issues worsened and a favorite brand of expensive concealer mocked me when I couldn't afford it. (Instead, I did silly things like pay tuition.) I returned a lot of cosmetic products and honed my negotiation skills to wisely use what little money I did have to spend on makeup.

When friends started getting married, I was there with makeup in hand to make them look flawless and perfect. Others started asking what I charged. What? You could make *money* playing with makeup? I was hooked. This was way better than actual work. Then I found SeneGence cosmetics in 2001, a line of skin care that actually worked for my lifelong skin issues, and that's not all: the makeup stayed on all day. Literally, my brides couldn't kiss it off, and there was no smudging. I was able to make my full-time living in the beauty world, loving every minute of it. Until then I hadn't been trained or certified by anyone other than my own artistic eye. Then, while at an expo outside of Boston showing the skin-care/makeup line I loved and sharing my makeup application tips, I was offered a position at a local beauty school teaching the advanced makeup class. That's when I knew this makeup thing wasn't just a fun job; it was my unique gift to share with others.

When the opportunity to actually become certified as a makeup artist came, I took it, realizing I had been a makeup artist for years. I had always been a good artist—and as a teenager during the makeup counter debacle, I had figured out that she was just using a different kind of paint. I may not have liked her interpretation of my face, but at least she showed me the power that a few tubes of color could have. My love of art gave me courage to see what I could do. The first time I got paid significant money to put makeup on someone, my knees shook, hoping she would like it. She did.

The first rule of makeup is: be willing to try. You will never get good at putting it on if you don't experiment with different techniques. You know you better than any expert. Honor your coloring. The intensity of color is dictated by your personality. If you are a bold personality you can go darker. If you are more timid, lighten up the color regardless of what trends say. I wear bright red lip color because it makes me look hot. If you are not sure, start with the less-is-more rule and blend as you go.

Makeup is not rocket science. There are no PhDs in makeup. You get good by playing with it. As far as that first makeup goal of mine—to not be made fun of—I've learned other ladies are too busy worrying whether they look okay to really worry about how you look. Learn a few simple rules and you will do fine. Don't worry if you make a mistake. It's not a tattoo—it comes off with makeup remover. (Since this is too hard to put in words, there are visual step-by-step tips for different makeup looks on my blog.)

Skin Care

Caring for your skin is important; it's as simple as that. And after decades of studying and experimenting with skin care, I can affirmatively say it does go a long way toward assisting and preserving our beauty, but don't ever think you're getting a miracle in a bottle. Advertisements lead us to believe it exists—an instant face-lift, prevention of stretch marks, baby-soft smoothness, acne-free skin in three days, reversal of the aging process, a special cream for every problem. Certain products can help offset problems and enhance your skin. (I mention my favorites on my site.) However, factors like genetics and aging are part of the formula of our skin. The aging process is a natural (and beautiful) process that happens to all of us. Acceptance, not denial, looks better on everyone! A smile not only lifts your spirits but also adds a glow to your face. There is nothing wrong or ugly about aging unless it is done with a scowl. When working with a client, I want her to look great for her age, not distort her until she doesn't look like herself.

The younger you are when you learn proper skin care, the greater the payoff later in life. If you are good to your skin, it will be good to you! Eat right, drink water, get sleep, cover up in the sun, and moisturize. Your skin is your body's largest organ; it is a reflection of your overall health.

Tips for a Good Skin-Care Routine

As you mature, your skin gradually becomes thinner and often drier. Moisturize inside and out! Drink lots of water and find the right product to moisturize your skin, particularly in drier climates. Select the proper products for your skin type. Use the treatment for your skin that best works for the way your skin is behaving. Skin is very fragile, and tissues can be easily damaged; use your ring finger and middle finger when applying skin care products because they are your weakest fingers and will be the most gentle. Who knew that your little pinky was so tough?

Millions of people use the same soaps and lotions to take care of their faces as they do the skin on their bodies. The face requires unique and specialized care and gentle products. Try the following steps for a clean, fresh, awesome you. (There are more in-depth tutorials on this topic on my website, but here's enough to get you started.)

Cleanse Your Face

The first step in the skin-care process is to cleanse your face. The purpose of a cleanser, or facial soap, is to gently remove dirt, debris, germs, grime, excess oils, and leftover products on your skin. Cleanse your neck also. This is often the first area to show signs of aging. Proper cleansing not only removes impurities but can also feed the skin proper nutrients through increased blood flow. Wash your face twice a day, morning and night—night is the most essential. Use lukewarm water and a mild cleanser. Stay clear of harsh soaps, detergents, alcohol, and other irritants that can harm the skin. Be careful not to cleanse too often, because it can damage or dry out your skin.

Start with a warm, wet face, splashing several times with warm water at the sink or in the shower. When your skin is warm, the pores open so they can be more completely cleaned out. Pores that are not properly cleaned harden with yucky stuff in them. Don't sleep with yucky in your pores. Please.

Once your face is warm and wet, use your fingertips to dab cleanser all over your face. Never use a washcloth; it's like rubbing sandpaper on wood. Just like brushing your teeth, proper facial cleansing cannot be done in a couple of minutes. Massage away the grime and dirt that has collected on your skin during the day. Gentle massage is key; never pull or tug at your face while applying a product.

Splash warm water on your face a couple times until your face feels free of residue. Then air-dry or pat your face with a clean towel.

Moisturize

Finally, moisturize; make sure your face remains slightly moist while you apply the moisturizer. The basic law of beauty is that everyone, no matter what gender or skin type, should moisturize. Even if your skin is oily, it will benefit from moisturizer. Even if you have acne, use moisturizer—just make sure you use products designed for acne; the wrong moisturizer will seal oil into your skin like plastic wrap.

How much should you moisturize? Your skin will tell you. When your skin is tight, it's crying out for moisture. If your skin is burning, it is asking for more moisturizer. If you add more moisturizer and your skin still burns, stop using it and find a moisturizer with a smaller molecular structure that can penetrate your skin.

Don't just slap moisturizer on; massage and listen to your skin. Apply a light coating to smooth any roughness, refining your skin to make a great surface over which to glide your makeup—which will help you blend the foundation to perfection.

These three steps take only two minutes to do. If you do them twice a day, you will see a noticeable difference in your skin's smoothness and integrity. There will be fewer blemishes and dry spots, and you will find that there will be days you will want to go without makeup because your skin looks so great.

I'd like to give you an analogy that I share with my clients; I think it helps make sense of skin care. Hidden deep within your skin, at its very base, is a general. Like most generals, he is hanging out where it is safe—next to the supply line (blood that carries nutrients) and far away from the onslaught of the front lines.

The general is directing his soldiers according to their rank and purpose. On the front line are the pawns of the army—the infantry. They are subject to all the new ideas you try to fix your skin; you scrub, peel, and burn off the top soldiers. The soldiers next in line, those just behind the fallen comrades, throw up their shields, terrified and peeing their pants. The front line, reduced in number, is scared smooth in appearance. The general is confused—but being a man of action, he makes a decision to send up more reinforcements (oil).

Just because the skin looks smooth doesn't mean the skin is actually healthy. Surface appearance is not the sole thing to look at when determining the health of your skin. Semiregular spa treatments will not give you radiant skin any more than working out once a month will give you flat abs. It's the little things you do every day that make or break your skin. Love on your skin daily. Your skin doesn't live in the utopia of the rainforest. Instead, it is being barraged by free radicals, smog, your co-workers' sicknesses, and children who think you are a human Kleenex. It's critical that you cleanse and moisturize it to its happy place.

Ingredients are important, but don't look exclusively for all-natural or organic products. Too often, those labels have become sales tactics. After all, fecal matter is also all natural. And renewable. Look for ingredients and products with independent lab results, not just sales slogans. Look for ingredients designed to nourish the skin and make a difference in the health of your skin.

This should go without saying, but never take skin-care advice from someone with bad skin. That is like asking someone who has never been married how to have a lasting, enduring marriage. All they can give you is theory. Look for results. And remember: Products don't work by osmosis from the bottle; you actually have to use them on your face. And many products take weeks to show whether they work, because your skin has renewal cycles you have to patiently wait through. (If you need more details in order to put together your look, don't stress out. You can find more in-depth information and visual examples on my blog or through my workshops or personalized makeovers. You can find me at yourglamourconnection.com and letagreene.com.)

Above all, remember that there is more to you than just a great wardrobe or a pretty face. You need to take care of your whole body, inside and out. Be kind to yourself. Be patient with your body and take good care of yourself for the benefit of your health and for those who depend on you. Get enough sleep; it will not only help your hormones regulate better, but connecting with others in an awesome way is easier when your brain is awake. The term *beauty sleep* is real— not just for outer beauty, but also for a kind disposition. As you take care of "all" of you, your look will fall into place and you will be healthier and happier. And hotter!

Hotness Challenge

This chapter provided step-by-step instructions for a critical kind of makeover. No, I'm not referring to the section about makeup. Or the stuff about skin care. Or even the Power Notebook—good as all those things are. I'm talking about your *closet*.

For this Hotness Challenge, I want you to start by pulling every little last thing out of your closet and heaping it on your bed. Then pull out the vacuum and the dust cloth and anything else you need to give your now-empty closet a good deep cleaning.

This challenge doesn't include getting the stuff back in your closet. Instead, it takes you through a great exercise in figuring out *what* needs to go back in the closet. With all your things heaped on your bed, pick up one item at a time. Here's your challenge with each one:

1. Figure out if it still fits. If you haven't worn it in the last month or so, put it on now. Do seams pull or strain? Is it bunched up anywhere? Do buttons gape? Or, on the other side of the coin, is it too large? Unless you're an accomplished seamstress and know you'll do alterations in the next week or so, toss it. (I know a woman who lost quite a bit of weight and, not wanting to get rid of a favorite skirt, hung on to it from one season to another

for *eight years* before finally admitting she didn't want to take it apart and reconstruct it.)

2. If the item still fits, try to remember the last time you wore it. If you haven't worn it in the last year, toss it.

3. If the item still fits and you've worn it within the last year, determine how happy it makes you. *What?* Clothes can make you *happy?* Absolutely. Does it make you feel like a million bucks when you wear it? Do people compliment you when you wear it? Do you find yourself smiling as you slip into it? Is the color one that you love? Does the style flatter you? If so, keep it. If not, toss it!

If you've done your challenge well, you're left with a pile of stuff on your bed that fits, that you like enough to wear fairly regularly, and that makes you happy. Follow the rest of the suggestions in the chapter on how to *organize* all that stuff as you put it back in your closet, assured that you have the foundation for a wardrobe that enhances your hotness.

Just an aside here, but a very important one: when I say *toss it*, I don't mean dump it into a trash can. If something is badly stained, torn beyond repair, or just plain offensive (though you wouldn't have put anything like that in your closet to begin with), then maybe it deserves a one-way ticket to the city dump. Otherwise, there are many places that gladly accept (and usually desperately need) gently used clothing and shoes. Consider a local women's shelter, charity shop, or even a friend or acquaintance. You'll end up with a closet that functions well *and* the satisfaction of brightening someone else's life—a real boost to hotness!

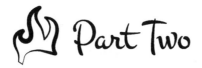 *Part Two*

NOW THAT YOU'RE HOT
FINDING OR REDISCOVERING YOUR PERFECT MATCH

*Where there is love
there is life.*

—MAHATMA GANDHI

Chapter Nine

―――――――― ❧ ――――――――

FINDING PRINCE CHARMING
IS HE *HOT* ENOUGH?

WINNIE was my mother's school teacher. Winnie loved my mother and regularly mentored her. But more significant, she believed in my mother, constantly asking what she was reading or what her dreams were. She offered love without judgment and taught without criticism—things my mother never got at home. When Winnie got older, she could no longer live alone, and my parents invited her to come and live with us. Winnie became my much-loved grandma of my heart.

Winnie taught me many things too—among them how make award-winning cinnamon rolls. She taught me how to spread thick dabs of butter on the dough and how to sprinkle on cinnamon and sugar, adding just a little more than I thought I should because in the heat the butter and spices mingled with each other—which was what made them so good. She taught me how to cut the rolls with a thread so I didn't pinch the dough together and so I could make uniform, perfect rolls.

Nothing was sweeter than being handed a cinnamon roll from Winnie because her rolls also came with a listening ear. Nothing Winnie did was for show; I can't even imagine her doing something to impress others. I felt love around her; it tasted like cinnamon and smelled like her body powder, fresh and clean. Love touched my face and encouraged me.

She was my roomie when I was a little girl; we shared a queen bed in the basement. The chicken coop was outside our window, and she said their sound reminded her of the farm on which she grew up. Her loving hands and her gentle, wrinkled touch have stayed with me even though she died when I was just eight.

Winnie was legally blind, but the only service she asked from us was to read to her. I am sure my reading at that age was more of a service from her to me as she took the cues from my sounds to help me say the word for which I was searching. I usually read the simple stuff, not Shakespeare. At the time, Winnie was the oldest student to ever attend Brigham Young University; she was studying anthropology and archeology. She taught me that the most profound difference you can ever have is impacting the heart of someone else. She has been gone for thirty years, and I can still remember how her love felt. She gave it freely, without judgment.

Though I didn't know it at the time, having Winnie in my life prepared me in many ways for one of the most sublime experiences in my life: finding my Prince Charming. Without consciously realizing it, I was hoping to find someone who would make me feel just as loved as she did . . . someone who would give me that love without judgment. And after kissing lots of frogs, I finally found that person . . . the prince for whom I had been looking.

But before I could marry the dashing and charming Mr. Greene, I had to meet his family. I assessed them as much as they assessed me. They were seeing what kind of addition I would make to the family, and I was seeing what their family dynamics were. Nathan is one of six kids. He is the oldest son but the last to find his true love. He had left home at barely seventeen, having gotten straight As with only one A- in high school, a fact he finds a little embarrassing. Just to equally share, I graduated with honors—barely (3.54)—and I am proud of this. He went on to school with both an academic and

ROTC (military) scholarship. He majored in electrical engineering and minored in math, physics, and Spanish. He is my sexy nerd (a term he doesn't really love . . . sorry, love).

The Spokane home in which his family was raised had one tub and two toilets; the second of those was added by my future father-in-law in what was then a closet. My mother-in-law-to-be was an avid decorator, and each room had a theme. I could see that Nathan wouldn't be bothered by my decorating dreams since he had already been broken in by her. She kept a clean home. His sisters were all beautiful, and smaller than me—that was my first disappointment, as my plans to let myself go would have to be abandoned (just kidding). Squeezing six kids, spouses—or their intendeds—and a couple of babies into the family living room was a challenge, but they had done this before. My future mother-in-law had coordinated everything. As we got down to eating, the family banter began.

Nathan's sisters were disgusted by the thought that he had been kissed. You'd expect some of that, but it went on and on, like he wasn't allowed to have someone show affection toward him. They didn't know what to do with how I behaved toward him—you know, like engaged people. Never mind anyone being happy for him. And that wasn't the only odd thing I noticed. No one was acknowledged for anything brilliant, thoughtful, or helpful they had done. Every one of them had put effort into the meal; they had all worked together. But the family culture was interesting—no one was complimented for their good work in any area.

Later, when I discussed this with my husband, he said his parents didn't want to make the other kids feel bad if one of them accomplished something. As the years have gone by, this dynamic has amazed me all the more. All of my husband's family members are great people. Each is accomplished in his or her own way. To me, compliments and kind words are not a limited scarcity. You can pass them out equally and endlessly. Sitting there at dinner that day, there was so much to compliment. And I felt blessed to join a new family, but I knew this dynamic was not going to work for *my* family—the one I planned on creating with my future lover. And then I said it— *lover*. He was going to be my lover; we would make babies. But it might have been better if I'd just thought it instead of saying out loud, "Future lover, could you pass the potatoes?" The family looked at me with expressions you can now guess, and in mock surprise, I said, "What? He is!" And a new title for Mr. Greene was born. *Lover*.

When you approach the decision of who to marry, you have to take into account the family culture your lover will be bringing with him. My hubby-to-be had grown up with no acknowledgment as to all he'd strived to do and be, and it had resulted in pain and subconscious training in a certain communication style. Where we come from makes us the people we are. I knew his family had taught him many good and important things, but that experience also made me aware of the hurt he had inside and the work we'd have to do to avoid more hurt in our family. We could have muddled our way through things with miscommunication and bruises from our past baggage, but we decided to honestly face what we'd both come from and not let that determine our future. Right then and there I determined that our future family culture would be overflowing with positive words. I would treat my hubby as though he was the king of his castle.

And guess what happened? I did treat him like a king. And I got treated like a queen! (And yes, this required lots of work and there were setbacks, but we were both committed to *our* plan for *our* family.) And now I tell my daughter, Ailsa, that someday she will meet a man who is her prince and he will treat her like his princess, and they will get married in a beautiful castle and together they will be a king and a queen who will build a kingdom (home) for their own princesses and princes. I have my happily ever after—not because life is perfect but because I choose to see life as a cherished gift, as something to be savored, and as something to deliberately create. I choose to be happy. The secret to happiness is not getting everything you want; it is to be content with what you have.

So, how do you find your prince? In most princess stories there is a force that is seeking to hurt the princess. This force—the person I call He Who Is Stinky—is real. He will seek to enter any door not guarded by your determination. As young women, just as we are beginning our grand adventure, the stinky one will suddenly jump out, startling our beautiful horse, disrupting our hair. We could be knocked off our horse and have to wield our sword. I studied karate for six years. Every girl should be armed with the knowledge that she can kick Stinky's butt. By staring Stinky in the face, she knows she can resist his lies, manipulations, and favorite weapons. Don't fool yourself into thinking that your prince will save you regardless of the peril that surrounds you.

Stinky doesn't fight us head on; he looks for our weakness. His favorite with girls and women is to tell us that we are not worthy of our royal crown—that we are just a scullery maid. But so was Cinderella, and many other future princesses who realized their current job did not limit their capacity. Sometimes you may think you have met your prince, but you find out he is just a frog. Know that you don't have to kiss all the frogs to find your prince.

My first date was to homecoming. He was cool and on the football team. I was not cool or on the football team. I was flattered, and he knew it. As we danced, his hands slid to my backside, making me so uncomfortable that I wouldn't dance with him anymore. He mocked me. I felt dumb—and then he even tried to kiss me! I felt hurt. Did he only ask me out because he thought he could get a few cheap thrills?

I realized that the only thing I knew about him was that he was "cool." So after that, I made a list of qualities that boys had to have if they wanted to go out with me. At first it had just two things on it: take school seriously and believe in God. If a boy hated school then he probably didn't know how to apply himself enough to see that he would need to work one day, and he should probably learn how to do that. I didn't date a guy on his grades; I dated him on his effort.

This meant that boys who sluffed school were off the candidate list. If he swore, he was off the list. Admittedly, I was not the typical teenager—I was already working hard to contribute to my family and to buy the things I needed. Having bought my own car, clothes, and other necessities, I was not looking to marry a guy who didn't work hard too.

What? I was thinking about marriage in high school? No, I was gathering an idea of what kind of character I wanted to eventually marry. That's a key factor: *character*. Work on your character so that you can recognize the same effort in others. You will start to care less about perfect locks of hair because his character will be more attractive. After all, ladies, do we want to be loved for our perfection of body or character?

We ogle after the famous because of looks or the ability to sing or act but ask nothing about their character. What's wrong with being attracted to the good guy? Bad boys are kind of bad, and, well . . . they are not good. Oh, you think you can fix him? Save him from his badness? Think that if he loves you he will be good? If you want to fix something, ladies, pick up a hobby. Don't date and don't marry projects. Date and marry *finished products*.

Don't wait for the perfect product, because that just doesn't happen. Just make sure that the things you have to overlook are quirks, not character flaws! Remember the tried-and-true saying, "Anything that you dislike before marriage will bother you ten times more after marriage." Another classic line is, "Before marriage, have your eyes wide open; after marriage, put on your blinders." Blinders are used to keep a horse focused on his task and to keep him from wandering to other . . . umm . . . pastures. Figurative blinders help you focus and see just what you choose to see. I am glad that my hubby chooses to see my lovely body and not that flabbiness I will not confirm nor deny exists.

Oh, you say there are no good guys to date? Really? *None?* Not a single one? Trust me and a billion other married women: being married is not the goal—being married *well* is! You only need one guy to marry—not thirty-four. Learn to recognize this so you can recognize him—even if he is not as cute as your teen icon.

Okay. Let's get back to the list I made after that disastrous homecoming dance. My new rules limited the pool of boys I would date, and word must have gotten around. Even though others didn't know what was on my list, they knew I had one—and the guys who asked me out treated me like a princess. Never did I have another guy even try to grab my bum. Until my wedding pictures!

I especially remember one young man who asked me out. He was a year younger—and, as you all know, a year is *ages* different in high school. He was shorter than me, but I was five nine, so a lot of boys were! He worked hard. We were in a biology class together; perhaps he noticed me over the frog dissection. In all honesty, puberty was hitting him hard; he had sweat rings, and he dressed kind of, well, not cool. But he fit my list. So I said yes. It was to be his first date. He picked me up in a car that he had worked on himself, he was attentive to me, he was kind, and we had a great date. Yes, the dance pictures look like I am dating my younger brother, but neither he nor my brother tried any fast moves. He treated me like royalty. We remained friends. Why wouldn't we? Nothing awkward or embarrassing happened. After that date we did group stuff like sledding, and we went to the movies a couple of times; again he pulled no moves—he was a perfect gentleman.

Years later I was in the mall in my hometown. Hearing my name yelled out in a deep voice, I turned to see this amazing figure of a man coming at me. He was massively muscular. I had to remind myself that I was engaged (not yet to Mr. Greene) and was not supposed to notice his perfectly framed arms swooping me up with ease—not something commonly done by men, as the last time I weighed one hundred pounds was well inside elementary school. He kissed me soundly on the cheek and announced to the assembled gaggle of girls that I had been his first date! I nodded my confirmation. He proclaimed that he had been a nerdy geek; I thought it best not to confirm this. The girls mumbled things like, "No way!" He said I had taught him to date—that I was the best date ever!

Ladies/girls, there is a lesson in this: be nice to the young men, men that may be a little thwarted in puberty, because one day they will grow into themselves—and if they have been working on their character in their awkwardness, then they will also be men of character with looks to match their awesome internal nature. They will be dashing and handsome because the same thing happens to them that happens to us when our positive thinking increases our inner hotness and makes us all the more ravishing! As I like to say, I am not nearly as cute as you think I am—it is just my inner hotness radiating out.

Now, my fellow princesses, you need to know that women of character and hotness are extremely irresistible to lazy trolls. They "troll" around, looking for a young lady to fetch for them. In college a young troll found me attractive. He waited outside my classes, and though he was very attentive to me, he didn't fit my list. He was still trying to "find himself," and finding himself included not working on *improving* himself. So he was driving a nice car that he bought with his college money, and he was working a minimum-wage job instead of going to school—but he was *finding himself*. Problem was (for him), I was not looking to be found by someone who was lost.

One day, after weeks of his attention, I became totally frustrated and said to him, "Why do you keep coming around when I give you no encouragement?"

His reply? "Because I know you are strong and will carry me through life."

Wow! Can I say it again? WOW! Marry a finished product, not a project. Don't marry a man who is lazy in building his character no matter how attentive or cute he is or how relentlessly he pursues you. Whatever the packaging, he is a lazy troll—trolling for a woman to *have,* not to cherish; a woman he can possess.

I owe a great debt to my first boyfriend, Eric Spotted Elk, who respected my boundaries and taught me that men could be trusted. I hadn't always known that. A man who was something of an uncle to me used our relationship to hurt me in terrible, evil ways. Over many years, he worked to entrench his ideas into my thoughts, grooming me to accept his offenses to my body and soul as he sexually abused me. He made me feel that I was the one to blame, not him, and that secrecy had to be maintained to protect me. When he began all this I don't know, but learning in the quiet moments of my soul that God knew me gave me the courage and the words to remove him from my life. It was some time before I could find the trust to tell others who would have protected me. To those of you who know this pain, you know that evil wears a kind mask; it's not always clear to see, and only through the light of God can the outlines of evil be clear. Let me give you my sure knowledge that God loves you; please go find that for yourself. You are a daughter of God and your body is sacred. Never let a man/boy push you into doing anything you do not want to do. A boy may say he loves you so you should have sex. That is not love.

Instead, find a boy who fits your list. One of the best rules that has served me well is the 3/5-year rule. If five years ago he didn't meet your list, or he wasn't the man you wanted to be a role model to your children, fine—five years is a long time and a lot can change. *But*, if he has not met your list for at least the last *three* years, then you need to look elsewhere. Before he met you was he willing to be the prince you had been waiting for? Does he have the character you admire? This goes two ways—are you being the princess who is being prepped to be a queen? If you are working on your own character, you should get a man who has been working on his.

Compromise is a part of any successful relationship, but use compromise for things like where to put the sofa or where to go to dinner, not issues of character. For me, a man that goes to church weekly on his own was part of my list. I wanted a man I could pray with, worship God with, and with whom I could raise children. I didn't want to fight about faith. I also didn't want to hope and pray that my husband would go to work. I dated men who were hard workers in all kinds of professions and at all income levels. I was dating to find the right qualities of character—not a specific income level and not just that happy feeling in my toes. A lady I cleaned for once asked me if I was intellectualizing dating too much. I said, "Absolutely! You have to get past my head to have a chance at my heart!"

When a young man who didn't fit my list asked me out, I told him about my rule. Many boys thought it was a dumb rule, but it was my rule. That proves my point. They thought rules were dumb. I don't. I think *good* rules are great. To the young, real freedom means no rules, no restrictions—but those movies always end with explosions of some kind. They don't make movies out of the kind of romance I am talking about because there isn't enough conflict! The movies where the opposites attract—the princess and the thief, the vampire and the girl next door—create unions that are full of drama, which is why they make entertaining movies. But what is wrong with falling in love with a good, steady guy? Where is the drama? The danger? Trust me, life will give you drama—why knowingly create it? Life is hard enough even if you marry the right kind of person; why make it harder by marrying the wrong kind of person? Thinking about what you want before you fall in love will help you fall in love with the right person.

You are in control of your own destiny, my fair princesses. To us queens who find our king not as charming as he was as a prince—ask yourself what emotions you are focusing on. Which feelings do you feed? Don't bash men. Don't hang out with women who bash men. How long will it take before you are irritated about the same thing? I was given some wonderful advice as a newlywed from Cynthia, a dear friend of mine. She said, "Be known as a kind wife." How true! Over our marriage my husband has heard the words I have said behind his back; I was so glad they were kind. I sure love hearing what he says behind my back! If they are *not addicted* to drugs, porn, or suffering from some major dysfunction, men have very simple needs—food and the other thing. I am not saying they are stupid; I am just saying that as a group, men are not as complicated in what they need to be content as women are. Give them these two things, kindly and consistently, and they will fight to protect you and become your knight in shining armor!

Sexual purity is not an outdated idea. When a man's needs are met without commitment, why should he commit? Why step up to the responsibility to financially provide for a family? It is considered old-fashioned to cling to the idea of the traditional family. Divorce rates in the United States are around 50 percent, but that doesn't mean that every marriage has equal chances of breaking up. You can strengthen your marriage before you even get married by how you prep for it. Most of the experts agree that the following increase your chances of divorce:

Too young when married
Living together before getting married
Parents were divorced
Not having children
Death of a child
Low education
Low income
No religion
Abuse of alcohol or drugs
Pornography
Insecurity

Whoa! Being insecure! It is not a bad idea to work on being kind to yourself so that you can strengthen not only your own happiness, but the happiness of those who depend on you (your hubby and kids).

It's a well-known fact that you can read statistics almost any way you want, but the factors listed above were on almost every list of the causes of divorce.

Because we are human, every marriage, every relationship, has conflict. Learning how to deal with that conflict will make the difference of a good thing not going bad. Think of a relationship like raw meat. How do you treat meat? Do you leave it out for days? No, it would go bad and make you sick. A good relationship—marriage, friendship, or family—needs to be kept from spoiling by keeping off the "bacteria," the thing that will grow and fester and destroy the good of the relationship. That bacteria can't just be cut off—it has to be treated. It is best if it can be prevented from growing there in the first place.

When cooking meat, quick, intense heat holds the flavor in; heat that is too high for too long makes the meat tough and hard to chew. Cooking meat slowly makes it tender. I am always sad when I watch a movie in which the boy meets the girl, and in the next scene they are kissing passionately and taking off their clothes. The heat is so high, so intense, that they don't take the time to really create a long-lasting heat. The expectation is that the first of passion will always burn on full throttle—but the truth is that people who need that kind of fire are soon on to another flame.

Now that we understand how heat works in a relationship, let's get back to conflict. When in conflict, we are quick to respond and often say or do what we wish we hadn't. When you feel like you must respond and know you shouldn't, your situation is what I call "sticky." You are in the middle of a conversation and you feel like it has gone wrong. You are not sure why, but you're feeling stuck, uncomfortable, and, well, "sticky." When that happens to me, I don't respond to the flow—I step out of the situation. If I have to, I just say, "I feel sticky."

In the movie *Joe versus the Volcano*, Meg Ryan's character, being somewhat not bright, says, "I have no response to that." She is completely deadpan—something I find to be profoundly funny. Sometimes we just don't have a response. We were not prepared to hear that information. So why respond? When you are feeling sticky and say something anyway, you often step in something cruddy. And regardless of who put the cruddy mud there, it is now on your favorite shoes, and you are going to have to clean that sticky, stinky mess off.

If we can walk away in a spirit of forgiveness, we can leave and the mud kind of works its way off. But sometimes we need to stick around and work to clean things up. When we don't forgive we stay stuck where we are, a place where we will only attract more mud and crud. Have you ever made a mud pie? After making a few you decide you have to add some other ingredients: grass, berries, flowers, sticks, random hot wheels your brother left in the sandbox. If you leave the gooey, muddy mess out in the sun it becomes hard. Straw and mud were the original ingredients of the bricks that were used to build shelter. Adding other things made the mud a stronger brick. The same thing happens with our mud—the more we add to it and the longer we leave it out, the harder it becomes. Soon, we have a sturdy brick to add to the mud wall that shields us from everyone else. If you are feeling sticky, leaving your mud to harden by not communicating will only hurt you.

Unfortunately, there are mudslingers. They love to sling mud, then point to you and say, "Look, there is mud!" It is embarrassing to suddenly be looked at by the crowd with mud on the side of your face. To prove your innocence, you may be inclined to throw the mud back, but then you also become a mudslinger. How do you know if you are a mudslinger? Everyone else is at fault but you. How can you deal with mudslingers? I recommend a plastic shield—they are agile enough to move when you see the mud coming, and you can still smile at the mudslinger. Christ called this turning the other cheek—forgive and move on. Let them keep throwing the mud. The other way to deal with mudslingers is to get out of reach.

One of my workshop attendees once suggested a third option for dealing with mudslingers: don't be a target. Wouldn't that be great if we could just get people to like us! Oh, but we can't—we can't fix others. If what you are doing is right—if it honors you, those who depend on you, and God—things may go your way some of the time, like they did for me when I set my dating standards and others respected me for it, but more often than not, others will in all likelihood fling mud at you until you stop living life at full awesomeness! You are a target if you are being amazing because crabby people don't like that. Life is not a popularity contest; it is a test of our character.

Character is the most important thing you can look for in a relationship. Alcoholics Anonymous was created when two men realized that an individual could not really overcome addiction to alcohol without the help of God. A passage called "The Serenity Prayer" is the foundation of the whole program:

> *God, grant me the serenity to accept the things I cannot change, The courage to change the things I can, And wisdom to know the difference.*

Hi, I'm Leta. I'm not an alcoholic, but I *am* a recovering fixer. I thought I could fix any relationship, even ones in which the other person did not have character and did not want to cultivate it. I had to discover through my own recovery that I *can't* fix a relationship that only I want to fix! As women we have such a great capacity to love. This is great as wives and mothers. But giving that devotion before a commitment is returned will leave you with a broken and bitter heart, wondering if you just didn't love enough! A perfect relationship is not made up of two perfect people but two flawed people who are perfectly committed to each other. Disappointment and heartache come from any relationship where one person's expectation doesn't meet what he or she is getting from the connection.

I personally find it hard enough to work on me and being my best self; finding the energy to really judge someone else is exhausting and sucks me to empty. I have relationships that I have tried everything I could to improve, but relationships are a two-way street. Just as in a business, an assessment of the cost must be made. Is the output of time and resources worth it? The only relationships I am willing to give my all to are my husband and children. Sorry, but if you are a mudslinging crab, I will smile nicely at you from behind my plastic shield. In the past I have caused my hubby stress by trying to mend relationships that were extremely difficult and filled with drama because I wanted the relationship so much. I finally realized that while I wanted the relationship, the other person didn't—at least not nearly as much as I did. That person just didn't love or like me in the same way I loved and liked him or her. That didn't make the other person bad—it simply came down to different expectations. So I smashed the bricks that kept me locked into that location on that battle field and got out of flinging distance—preserving my own happiness and that of my family.

As women we seek love; it's in us to love. Men are fulfilled by career and action. We are fulfilled by security and connection. Both needs can be met when both people realize they are not perfect— that perfection is reserved for later. Then they can enjoy the process of becoming together.

So how do you find love? As you know, I am no lover of math, so it's a very big deal that I'm giving you a math analogy:

$$1 + 1 = 2$$
$$\tfrac{1}{2} \times \tfrac{1}{2} = \tfrac{1}{4}$$
$$1 \times \tfrac{1}{2} = \tfrac{1}{2}$$
$$1 \times 1 = 1$$

If you feel like this might be a letdown after the way I promoted it, just wait. Two people get married and they think that they will have their separate lives and separate bank accounts and can split if needed from the relationship. They figure if they fall out of love it's okay, because it's just two separate people in a legal contract.

And the halves? Think about that—people say it all the time. They go out looking for "their better half" to complete them and make them feel whole. NO ONE can make you feel full if you are only a half. If you are looking for someone else to make you feel good, complete, or happy, you will only become less. The hole will eat at you until you decide to fill it.

How do you fill it? Start deciding what you mean to God, what you mean to yourself, and what good can you do today. I loved my time as a full-time mom. I always worked, but when my children were young, I worked only a few short hours of the day. For me, being a mom—wiping their tears, hearing their sweet thoughts—was fulfilling because I knew, like Winnie, I was giving without judgment, giving without expecting to receive anything back. (Of course, I do expect slobbery kisses and handmade cards on Mother's Day!)

I find contentment as a wife and mother because long before I became a wife, I decided that my value as a daughter of God meant I was worthy of marrying a son of God. I decided that I was a person of honor. And once I made that decision, I tried to work on me. Sometimes I failed. Sometimes I made mistakes. But I refused to let those failures and mistakes define me. Instead, I looked in the mirror and began each day with hope that today I would get it right. At the end of the day I looked at how I'd done and worked to do better.

There isn't a seminar you can attend that will make you like you. It takes practice. It takes working on you, refining your thoughts, and making them better. You can only trust someone as deeply as they trust themselves, and you can only learn to trust yourself by loving yourself. Life is not about pursuing perfection or happiness; it is about pursuing character and honor. As you seek, those perfect moments will come, and happiness will be easy to choose. Even when things are hard.

Marriage is not about what you can get but what can you give. Only when one person who loves themselves is ready to wholly give themselves to another do you have a powerful marriage equation. God's idea of marriage is to become ONE—to be so united that He will multiply what you could be as one person, and you are enhanced as a powerful, combined, united force of being truly one.

Hotness Challenge

What's the most important thing you can do if you're on the lookout for your Prince Charming? Let me give you a tip: it's not to become the cutest girl in a five-county radius. Nope. The *most important thing you can do* is to decide you are of infinite value *long before* you even get close to letting some guy slip a ring on your finger. Why? Because if you're convinced of *your* value, you will consider for a marriage partner only a man who is also of value. No question—you'll know you're worthy of a royal crown, and you'll wait to take the plunge until someone can plunk such a crown on your head.

Here's a challenge that will help keep things in clear focus at a time when moonlit nights and heady cologne can tempt you to decide the crown's not that important:

1. Make a list of the qualities a man has to have in order to date you. (*Date?* That's right. Because at least in this country and at least in the last century, no girl has married a guy she didn't date first.) Think hard about this. This isn't the tall-dark-and-handsome list, though those are always nice. This is the *hard worker, optimistic, meets challenges with grace, never uses abusive language* kind of list. It's the list by which you can live for the next five or six decades, because if you're lucky, that's how long you'll be married. Spend a week making your list. Cross stuff out if you need to. Add as you should. By the end of the week, make sure you have a list that describes *your* Prince Charming—exactly the type of man with whom you want to spend the rest of your life.

2. You thought *that* was challenging? Ha! Here's the real challenge: By the time you reach the altar, *that list should describe you.* That's right. Become the type of person you want to marry—because I can guarantee you, *that's* what any prospective husband will find hot! So what if you have porcelain skin and a whittled waist! Life happens. Skin sags and waists fill out. But honesty and cheer and compassion and optimism never go out of style—and any guy worth having will know that. Work on your character. Use your list. Take pride in what you have to offer. After all, you're one hot commodity!

Chapter Ten

OWNING YOUR HOTNESS AND LETTING HIM OWN HIS
THE SECRET TO A HOT MARRIAGE

B EFORE WE GET DOWN to the brass tacks of discussing marriage, let's do a little review of the principles we've discussed so far—because they have particular application when you're trying to have a hot marriage. Marriage involves two people, and it requires the dedication of both to the principles that produce hotness.

Let's start with guilt. Guilt is there for a reason—it's there to teach us when we do something wrong. How we respond to that guilt can be very instructive. (We can sometimes feel guilt because of our cultural upbringing and not because we're actually failing to do the right thing, and sometimes even for situations in which we are actually victims—i.e., abuse victims often feel guilty—but since it's a complicated discussion to parse out, we'll focus on the simplest aspects that have to do with our healthy marriages.

When we feel justifiably guilty, we can do one of three things:

- Blame others
- Rationalize
- Make it right

Go back to what you learned in science and biology class. When cornered, animals will fight or flee. Well, we're animals too. No one likes to feel cornered or feel that he is wrong. But when we do realize we are wrong, what we do about it not only defines our character but demonstrates how we feel about ourselves. Interestingly, we project what we feel about ourselves onto the world—we believe that others are just like us, and we rationalize that other people are just as bad or just as good as we are.

When my children were three and five, I had the blessing of having two other kids in our home a few days a week. I loved them like my own kids. Their home life was very unstable. Their mother was charged with ninety-six counts of prescription fraud and was very open with her kids about her legal issues. I got a real snapshot into her rationalization when she told me the police were to blame for arresting her. They were "out to get her." She blamed everyone but herself.

The prescription fraud was just the tip of the iceberg. She also had an extensive history of check fraud, theft (including from us), health issues, $5 million in medical debt for which the taxpayers of our great country were paying—and, of course, she didn't work, so she was eligible for every single entitlement program. She took no responsibility for her health, financial situation, honesty, or the stability of her children. But wait! *Society* was at fault, not her! *She* was the victim in all of this.

Eventually, in one of the most difficult episodes of my life, the mother demanded that I give her $20,000 if I wanted to see her children again. Our family was heartbroken. We loved those children deeply and still miss them. The hardest part is to know that her example clouded out valuable lessons of integrity, honesty, and self-respect that her children could have learned from others.

We all come with knowledge of what is right and wrong, and life can be so brutally hard that we can have these tender feelings of truth squeezed out of us like vise grips on our soul. I believe in redemption. I believe that the Atonement of Christ redeems us from pain and from loss. Every one of us will fall short of what we know is our best; this is part of being human. But because every religion has a redeeming personage who helps us through the dark feelings of our own weakness, we need to accept that help and seek to improve our character. Our character is molded solely by us, and our impact on others is a reflection of our character. After a certain age, we are responsible for what we think and do. It is not someone else's responsibility to boost our self-esteem. Others cannot validate us into feeling good about us.

How you choose to think will not only dictate the pathways of your brain but will determine your overall mood. What you make a habit of focusing on will help you see what is really possible and not just what you feel like doing. We all do a lot of things we don't feel like doing. Why? Because those things are right. We don't always feel like getting out of bed in the morning, but we do. We likely don't love changing a dirty diaper, but we do it—and we usually do it with a good attitude because of the love we want to express to our little one. Each day is full of things to be done. With Vanity Prayers, the hope is that you will focus on why you are doing what you're doing and what your purpose is; instead of walking through your day as a victim who seems surprised that the sun came up once again, you will instead be living, loving, and ready to be amazing. It all starts in your own head! The impact of your thinking will influence everything in your life.

Change is hard because it is new. Realize that at first, even when the change is good, you may resist it. Others may not like it, and they may resist it too. To maintain the decision you have made, you need your WHY in place. If your WHY is greater than your discomfort at doing a new thing, you will push past the discomfort. Some gurus tell you to put a picture of a fancy home or car on your fridge and to visualize living in that house or driving that car. I don't think homes and cars really motivate us to be our best. Better than imagining a *thing*, imagine being *happy*. Crazy, huh?

When things felt dark for me as a young girl, I was given the advice to build my future. Habits—those impulses to do things we have always done or seen done—take real effort to change. It's not a matter of just filtering the messages that pop in our heads; we must replace those messages with something true.

A wonderful woman named Rita Debry (Hi, Rita!) gave me an analogy that has served me so well. It's such a good analogy that I share it with most of my clients. Now I'm going to share it with you. In life we are given a hand of cards. We have to pick up the cards and play in the game—we can't just throw down our cards and refuse to play. There's more: we can't decide when the game ends, even if we don't want to be in the game anymore.

That's it. You *are* in the game. If you don't like the cards you hold—your short temper, your lack of patience, your inclination to stretch the truth, your feeling that you are a victim—then change the card you don't like! How? Study people who hold the cards you want. What does the patient mother do? Ask her; learn. What heroes do you have? What did they do to overcome? Read what others have done to win with the hand they were dealt.

I am not the person I used to be. I am better. I don't say that I am better than anyone else; I am better than I USED TO BE. I have worked on me. I learned from others—not just people of history and famous icons but from the everyday heroes of my life: friends, family, neighbors, and church and business associates. In every arena of my life I have sought out mentors to teach me. Some of them knew they were mentors because I asked them questions; others were unaware of their impact on me because I watched them from afar, quietly observing and learning. It is a scary day when you realize that others are watching you, learning from you. What do you want to teach them? Are you willing to *actively* play your hand in the game of life?

Weeks before my sixteenth birthday, I found the car for me. I didn't choose it for its sleek design but for its price. What was a thing of beauty to me, my 1966 Dodge, was a joke to others. The girl from whom I bought the car sold it because it was just too big for her to handle. But because I had grown up with trucks, it was just right for me! Because the girl from whom I bought the car had a crush on my brother, Lance, she gave me some dating advice as she handed over the car. Talking about boys, she said, "You always have a choice." Those words hit me hard. *A choice?* I didn't feel like I had always had a choice. I hadn't chosen the circumstances of my life. I hadn't chosen to be abused. I hadn't chosen to have those I loved die. How could she say such a thing?

God has a way of speaking to us, even about things we don't want to hear. I had been praying, doing what I would come to call Vanity Prayers. I was working on my thinking. But I still saw myself as a victim, and I felt angry at her for unknowingly challenging that idea I had for myself. I *was* the victim! But here's where the life-changer comes in: Even though I had been victimized, I didn't *still* have to be the victim.

What happens to us is very different from who we are. Just as I am not defined by the bad that happens to me, I am also not defined by the good. I am not titles and accomplishments. None of us is. I believe the only thing we really need to know about ourselves is that we are children of God. Sadly, too often we seek our meaning from things, titles, jobs, looks—anything other than what really shows our true worth. The impact we have on other people is what shows us who we really are.

Sitting in the car that night, my fingers wrapped around the cold steering wheel, I knew it would go where I directed it. If I hit a brick wall, chances were it was because I guided it there. Earlier that same year I'd learned that I had to decide who I was; that night I learned I had to take control of the direction of my life. I had a choice. It was up to me. Bad and wrong things *had* happened in my life, but I had become a "victim" because of how I chose to react to those things.

It was not easy to realize that things may be 99 percent someone else's fault but that 1 percent was still mine to decide. What would

I do with that 1 percent? What decisions would I make with what
had happened? I had been a victim again and again because I had
not changed those things that made me a target. Considering the
girl I was, that was hard stuff for me to hear—and it was even harder
to implement the changes I knew I needed to make. It was a pivotal
decision to realize that I could choose. Later, when I read *Man's
Search for Meaning* by Victor Frankl, one of the most amazing books
ever written, I learned that regardless of where you are—even in
a concentration camp—you still have the power to choose. Were
the things I had gone through worse than being in a concentration
camp? Hardly! I find great comfort in knowing that my Brother,
Jesus Christ, knows my deepest hurts and has experienced greater
emotional and physical pain than I or any other person who has ever
lived could endure. He loves me. He loves each of us. He will listen
to us and offer His understanding, redemption, and hope.

What defines any of us is what we think, which leads to what
we do. What we do and why we do it is who we are as a person.
Others may misunderstand why you do something, and even with
the best of intentions you will make mistakes. We are not God. We
don't always see the long view. We make judgments without all the
facts. We assume, we bicker, we get hurt, and we respond, often
not in the best of ways. We are human. And with that comes the
need to forgive ourselves, learn from it, be better, and give others
the same freedom. We are never 100 percent right or 100 percent
wrong, and if you think you are . . . you're wrong. Think how that
applies to your marriage.

What impact do you have on others? That impact is a reflection
of what you think about, what you say. Those two combined are what
you project into the world. We project to the world the treatment we
expect from it. As a young girl I projected to others that it was okay
to hurt me, to be mean to me. And that is exactly what happened. In
sales, they call it *the posture*; in entertainment, they call it the *IT factor*.
It comes from within the person, and those around them read it and

make decisions about the person based on it. It cannot be faked; it is simply who they are. If we have determined that we are the victim, leaving the abuser won't solve the problem. Why? Because we've determined that we're the victim, so we will find another person to abuse—victimize—us. We operate where we are comfortable, even if it is a bad place. We won't change unless we consciously decide to become a different person. It is our decision. No one else can change you, just like you can't change anyone else.

Changing Him—Or Not

Let's look at how that applies to marriage. No one else can change you—you have to do it. And you can't change anyone else. At first blush that doesn't seem very fair. You change but he doesn't? But let's review the important point from above: You can't change someone else. If you've done your job and married a finished product, the time has come to appreciate it for what it is. You're in charge of your hotness and he's in charge of his.

Ladies, sometimes we are naggy hags who try to make over men so they will be . . . well, more like *women*. Yes, I made up the word *naggy*. It should be a word, just like *pooperness* should be a word. I hereby declare it a word. I may have a whole dictionary by the time I'm done. I can make up words because I'm a woman and my mind is already going a million miles an hour, which may be one reason we nag when men can't keep up. But men don't think the same way we do. They are not the same. This is part of why we like them and they like us—we are so fascinating to discover and to learn about.

As a newlywed, my husband did something I knew was wrong. Had I talked with my girlfriends about what he'd done, I could have made him look bad and me noble for putting up with him. Fortunately for my marriage, I took it to prayer instead of to my girlfriends. I knelt there in my living room and started my prayer by explaining why this was such a problem and why it had to be fixed.

As I prayed I looked up. On our living room wall hung a sword that my hubby had bought while living in the Canary Islands for two years. Being very visual, I focused on that sword and realized that God was teaching me that the sword cuts both ways—each side is used by the skilled swordsman to accomplish its purpose. If I were to remove the thing about my hubby that was bothering me, I would also be removing the good side of the quality—all part and parcel of the man I love. God has blessed me with a man who is very focused, determined, driven, and clear. Someone else may see these same traits as demanding or otherwise negative. But they are all things that attracted me to him. He is so clear. I know what bothers him, how he feels about something. There is no hinting, no layers to figure out. I know that he is steady. I knew when he asked me to be his wife that he meant it not just during a moment of passion but as a permanent commitment to love me, to serve me. He is a rock. I would never want to change that.

I realized while looking at that sword that I wasn't giving him the space he needed. I was about to pick him apart as though I had the surgical ability to do so—I was about to try to fix him. I changed my prayer that day. Instead of trying to fix him, I asked for help to fix my impulse to be a naggy hag.

No one wants to be with a nitpicking, naggy hag. Instead, I focused on praising him for his efforts, something that is easy to do when you're dating and falling in love but harder to do when you are building a marriage and a foundation for a life together. It's even harder when you find, in shock and horror, that your perfect groom has flaws! What torment would rain down upon him if he were to point out that his bride was less than perfection?

One of the best pieces of advice we were given at our wedding was to go to bed at the same time so we could pray together. This seems so easy, but he is a morning person, and I'm a night person. How many nights have I stayed up late to put on one more coat of paint when he had to get up at 5 A.M. for military PT? I love to decorate. He loves a modern style with clean lines. I love vintage finds. He puts up with me and even praises me for my efforts to beautify our home. We really are different people, but that doesn't mean we can't get along.

He is a get-it-done-in-segments, never-put-it-off, work-before-play person. I am a chew-the-whole-elephant-now, stay-up-and-get-it-done, dance-funky, and find-ways-to-make-work-play person. Writing this book couldn't be done in a day; it was years in the making. Fortunately, I have learned and observed from my husband that all worthy tasks cannot be completed in a day. Differences don't matter. Go to bed at the same time.

A couple of weeks after the sword incident (which would sound so gruesome out of context, wouldn't it?), as we finished our prayer my good hubby said, "I do (*the very thing I wanted to fix*) and I realize that it could be hard for others, and I do this because (*something that I didn't even see*)." In my impulse to fix him, the scripture came to my mind, "Or how wilt thou say to thy brother [husband, in my case], Let me pull out the mote out of thine eye; and, behold, a beam is in thine own eye?" (Matthew 7:4).

I could have pointed out to him the mote in his eye—more like a little sliver, really just a speck of wood—and been completely unaware of the beam, the big *honkin'* piece of wood coming from my own. Who wants a blind surgeon to perform an operation on them? There are times when we are so quick to see ourselves in the best light and others in the worst. Try giving others the trust that they are doing their best. Decide that there is enough work to do on directing your own thoughts, words, and actions that you don't have time to nitpick others. We have all been wrongly judged. Let us not judge others wrongly. Let's face it—even when given all the facts, we can be wrong. It can actually be funny how wrong we are!

Why is it that we think we see others so clearly? What do we think we know about our family, our spouses, that we don't really know? I had a neighbor one time who came over and yelled at me, accusing me of being a lazy mom because I didn't play with my kids; instead, he pointed out, I just sat watching them. What he didn't know was that my SI joint, which is part of the connection between the back and hip, was severely damaged due to the many miscarriages I'd had. Every step I took was painful; it literally took years of physical therapy for me to be able to walk without pain. He didn't see my subtle limp. It was hard to have so many things that I had once done so easily, like lifting, running, and even walking, be so difficult. I didn't tell him what he couldn't see, because he clearly didn't like me and nothing I could say would convince him otherwise. He saw what he saw. He thought he knew all about me when he really didn't know me at all.

As children we are natural sponges. That is why we learn so quickly to walk, eat, and speak—things that are actually complicated tasks. Our minds are actually more sophisticated and capable than any computer. They say we use only a portion of our brains—but like any body part, the brain must be engaged to be strong. Use your own brain to choose the hand you will play and be responsible for it. Don't blame anyone else. Your self-esteem is not based on the words or actions of others. They cannot validate you into you liking you. That is your responsibility. Yes, you will be judged and you will make mistakes. That is where forgiveness comes in. I would rather assume the best of my own potential and someone else's than the worst. The German philosopher Johann Wolfgang von Goethe said, "Treat a man as he is and he will remain as he is. Treat a man as he can and should be, and he will become as he can and should be." We all grow, and others can too. We should give them the ability to do so. We are not responsible for their growth, but we *are* responsible to not hold them back.

Your life is what you make it. You are in charge of you. You are not in charge of others. We are all messed up enough that working on you should take most of your energy! Focus on what you can change; focus on what you have control of: you and the attitude you choose! Decide today what card you will play with the hand you have.

Hotness Challenge

Want a hot marriage? Be a hot marriage partner!

Want to be a hot marriage partner? Remember this: Your spouse likely decided he wanted to get to know you based on how you looked—those first impressions are what make us want to come back for more. But that was a *long* time ago. Since then, he's definitely come back for more. He's learned how hot you are inside. He's figured out that your character is a lot more important than your hairstyle. He appreciates your values more than how white your teeth are. Sure, you still have to brush those teeth so he has a sweet-tasting kiss, but the things that make him want to keep kissing you are a lot more than skin-deep.

We just talked about how life is like a card game. You get dealt a hand of cards. But consider this: you can change the cards you don't want! Huzzah! Are you holding a *selfish* card? Throw it on the discard pile and trade it for a *generous* card. It works—and *you* hold the ability.

Here's how to end up with a hand that would make any gambler grin:

1. During the next week, keep a small notebook close at hand—on the kitchen counter, in your purse, in the glove box of your car. At least once each day, record in that notebook some of the cards in your hand. List the good, the bad, and the ugly. Your goal is to have a complete list by the end of the week.

2. On day 7, circle the good cards. Those are the ones you'll keep in your hand. *Happiness. Gratitude. Optimism. Loving nature.* You know the ones—the things that make people want to spend time around you.

3. Starting on day 8, start to work on the cards you want to discard. Place a check mark next to the crappy card you most want to discard. That doesn't mean you can get rid of only one card between now and the end of time—it means that you're more likely to succeed and achieve lasting change if you work on a single goal at any given time. After you've traded that crappy card for an awesome new card, you can start the process over if there are more icky cards in your hand.

4. Turn to a new page in the notebook. Write the name of your crummy card at the top of the page. Now write a few thoughts about why this is a crappy card. How does it impact your relationship with others? Has it hurt someone else? Has it hurt you? Is it holding you back in some fundamental way from the life you want to live? Be specific. The more specific you are, the better equipped you are to know *why* you want to change.

5. Next, write a few thoughts about how your life would be different if you were able to get rid of that card and change it for a great card. Really put some thought and effort into this. You're not allowed to jot down any quick clichés.

6. Finally, write the names of at least three people—people you personally know, people you've read about, public figures—who exemplify the new card you'd like to hold. Spend some time thinking about those three people and how you can become more like them in that particular quality. Jot down some ideas.

7. *Now for the most important part:* Use what you've written to write down one actionable goal you will work on

during a specific period of time to come closer to getting the card you want.

8. On day 9, start executing your goal! *Take action.* What matters is not that you win a race but that you gradually become better than you used to be. That you choose truth and happiness over falsehoods that held you back. That you cultivate the qualities that will make you a truly hot companion!

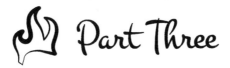 Part Three

HAPPILY EVER AFTER IS A CHOICE?
HOW TO KEEP THE NEW YOU GROWING HOTTER EVERY DAY

*The happiness that brings enduring worth to life is not
the superficial happiness that is dependent on circumstances.
It is the happiness and contentment that fills the soul
even in the midst of the most distressing circumstances.*

—BILLY GRAHAM

Chapter Eleven

---- 🖐 ----

THE ROAD ISN'T ALWAYS SMOOTH
STAYING HOT UNDER PRESSURE

MY SON'S NAME is Nathaniel, meaning "gift of God." He was my firstborn child but my sixth pregnancy. Albert Einstein said that insanity consists of "doing the same thing over and over again and expecting different results." But Mickey Rooney said, "You always pass failure on your way to success." I like to say that I am insanely successful. I do believe the trying is valuable; success is not just getting, but becoming.

I wanted to be a mother. Stealing other people's babies is frowned upon in society, and with my husband at the time serving in the military, we didn't have the resources to adopt. My husband decided to go to law school after serving in the military. I had started a business with SeneGence International the year before; I was doing well and loving that I finally got to play with makeup and art and design full-time. I had also worked as a medical interpreter for the deaf when I lived in Washington, DC—the city where Mr. Greene met me, fell madly in love with me, and asked me to be his wifey forever, and where I said yes!

Between the two careers I was confident that I would be able to support us, even though the cost of living was much higher in New Hampshire, where we would be headed for school. He would study;

I would work and dream that with *lawyer* attached to Mr. Greene's name, adoption would not only be possible financially but that we would be picked by the birth mother. Who wouldn't pick us?! We waved good-bye to dear friends in Oklahoma, ending that chapter of military service and heading off to the world of long hours, student loans, and . . . surprise!

The first week of school I found out my pregnancy was viable and Nathaniel would be joining us. I had four and a half months to figure out how I would be a mom while supporting our family financially. People who didn't know our history often asked if we regretted our timing with that pregnancy. I always replied that it is never a bad time for a miracle!

Nathaniel blessed our home beyond anything I could have imagined. Two miscarriages later, and Ailsa—meaning "promised of God"—joined our family during the last semester of law school. I would just like to brag for a moment. I put my hubby through law school while I was pregnant four times and gave birth to two kids. I just didn't want you to miss this, as it sounds a lot more glamorous than it was. Oh, wait—it doesn't sound glamorous? Hmmm, well I made it look good.

There were definite changes in my career path. I taught advanced makeup techniques in a beauty school and had women meet with me in my home during naptime so I could help them with their beauty needs. We lived on as little as we could so that I could be there for every coo, every smile, every fart, and every tear. I held Nathaniel's hands while he took his first steps. All the sacrifice—no vacations, no extras, no eating out, and tiny specks of Christmas—was worth it to be there when my kiddies needed me.

There I was, going through life, planning my actions, working for the best outcome. Life is not about controlling your life events or other people—it is about being in control of YOU! You can't control other people; trying to control others is manipulation and a great deal of pooperness! You can't control life, either. Things in life will hit you like a bus when you're least expecting it! *Really*, you might ask, *who gets hit by a bus?* Well, okay, maybe not a *bus*, but we all get hit by really large obstacles we didn't see coming. And when we do, it hurts!

On a typical Saturday morning you will find my hubby riding his bike; going fifty miles is no big deal to him. If the weather is bad he rides it in the basement on a trainer, a cycling thing that lets him "train" even in inclement weather. But in good weather he happily gets up at awful hours to ride while I stay in bed, safe and warm. As mentioned before, we all get hit by things, and on August 21, 2007, he was actually hit by a bus!

Literally. Hit by a bus.

It was a horrible phone call to receive. One of the passengers called me, and I could hear my husband's agony in the background. The bus driver had seen my husband and figured he could steer around him. He had plenty of space to go around my husband, and my husband was exactly where he should be. But the driver failed to make SURE he wouldn't hit my husband.

My hubby was thrown thirty-five feet; his scapula (shoulder bone) was broken on impact, and he tumbled through gravel that resulted in road rash over most of his body. His bike helmet was split open, so there was real danger of head injury and brain damage. The ambulance beat me to the accident; the decision was made to take him to the premier hospital in our area because of the possibility of brain injury.

It was a long drive. Having been a medical interpreter for the deaf in my early twenties, I knew how easily these amazing bodies of ours could get injured; I especially knew how fragile our brains were. What if my husband wasn't the same man? What if he was altered mentally from the accident? Alone in my car on the freeway, I repeated aloud what my marriage vows meant—not just if things worked out but through loss, miscarriages, buses, and brain damage.

His wonderful brain survived; the healing time was intense, but he is still him. For this I am thankful. I tell my children that when they were two and five, Daddy was hit by a bus and God let him stay with us. It's important to note that we did nothing to cause the accident. He was not playing chicken with buses and I was not driving the bus—it was a consequence of someone else's bad judgment. In the same way, a lot of the bad things that happen in life can be avoided by good decision-making, but life will still hit you, and it will hit you hard. This is because we don't live in heaven. We live on earth, and there are people here. Humans, once in a while, have been known to make stupid decisions. So if you are human, forgive yourself and forgive the other humans too—most of us are just trying to do our best.

Before the bus accident, I had been praying about how to grow my family. With nine pregnancies and only two kids under my belt, I knew that pregnancy didn't necessarily equal baby. I decided adoption was the way to go. I prayed about that, and the answer that kept coming back for me was no. I wondered why. It is not the purpose of this book to walk you through my personal heartbreak and the meanderings of my agony over my dysfunctional womb—I just want you to know that my sincere desire was to fill my home with the pitter-patter of little feet. One time a lady said that she could never adopt because she didn't know if she could love children who didn't look like her! *What?*! I pulled my two blond children to my side and said, "You love those you serve." Being a mother is not a picture-perfect world. It is messy, difficult, and full of smelly poo and slimy snot. If you want your child to look or be a certain way, then you're not ready to be a mom!

After my husband's bus accident my prayers turned to gratitude that the love of my life, my best friend, was still with me and our kids. I saw what I had instead of what I didn't have with more clarity. Though I was no longer praying for ways to expand my family, my husband and I learned through a deeply spiritual experience that God wanted us to get pregnant and that we were to trust in Him. Yes, medically we knew that didn't mean we should start decorating a nursery.

The next summer we were having a Fourth of July party with a few friends. The kids were playing games, the food was yummy, and I was very Martha for having a cake in red, white, and blue. The only bummer was that my hubby wasn't feeling well. We all know that chicks can carry on when feeling sick. The first time I got sick after my son was born I realized that never again would a sick day be as it had been—lying on the couch would no longer involve Jane Austen marathons or my favorite book. It would involve cartoons. But I have harbored the belief that a sick day for men is kind of great. After all, they have a woman doting on their every need. Don't get me wrong—I feel bad for my hubby when he is sick, but, honestly, when men get sick the tough guy sort of disappears, and they become a little . . . okay . . . maybe whiney.

That day, my hubby genuinely seemed to be pretty sick. I figured it was dehydration—he had gone on a long bicycle ride that morning—so I took him to the hospital. He was diagnosed with heat exhaustion. There we were in our little emergency department room; I was rubbing his back and trying to comfort him but was really thinking about my to-do list for the next day.

Suddenly he fell into my arms and died. I don't think it's possible to adequately explain how it felt to hold my husband's lifeless body in my arms. *Panic* may be the best word to describe it—*grief* seems too gentle to label the emotion that attacked me on a cellular level.

In that moment, God spoke to me, and I don't say that lightly. I heard words not from the outside, but from the inside. I know they weren't my own thoughts, because I was incapable of feeling or thinking anything beyond the torrent of fear surging through me. God was not speaking to my mind, which was in full freak-out mode. Instead, He was speaking to my soul—the soul that knows Him and can listen even when my logical mind tries to shut Him out.

What God told me in that emergency room is sacred and not to be read by others—but I will tell you that He said the kids and I would be fine. I felt a peace that was tangible. I could almost feel it physically not only calming me but instructing me. What I felt at that moment changed me. I can't *prove* that God exists, but neither can I deny that He is real. I know He is real with all my heart. It's a fact I know every bit as much as I know that I love my husband and my children. I still rely on faith when it comes to God's promises, but I *know* He is there.

That knowledge gave me the strength to not crumble in the corner of that emergency room—and, as it turned out, I would need that strength. I laid my husband down and looked at him. His face was like someone else's. What had made him *him* was gone. When someone dies, the soul departs and the body is left behind; without the soul, the empty shell of a body no longer looks familiar. I have often wondered if my husband's soul hovered above me, looking at his body and at his wife.

Evidently I shook him at that moment. And apparently I shook something loose, because he came back to life! The nurse walked in the room at that moment, and I calmly said, "He just died." She looked at both of us. He was dazed, and I had aged about twenty years in five minutes. She doubted my claim that he had died. I demanded an EKG (prior medical knowledge came in handy here). She reminded me that the EKG was very expensive, and this is when my hubby got a concerned look. I replied, "I don't care what it costs! I'm not leaving until I know why my husband just died in my arms!"

The nurse started hooking up the wires, looking at me the whole time like I was actually stealing funds from the hospital. She was reciting in a monotone voice the process of reading results when suddenly her tone changed. She ran from the room. Within what seemed like seconds, our room was full of medical personnel. She no longer doubted my account.

My hubby had suffered a major heart attack. His right coronary artery was completely blocked—in other words, half of his heart was not functioning. He'd been having little heart attacks all day without either of us realizing it; he'd felt nauseated, threw up several times, passed out once, and had pain in his arms, but was otherwise fine. The episode I witnessed is a kind of heart attack called the *widow maker* because 97 percent of people who have them don't survive. The doctors told us that a portion of his heart was now dead; they classified the damage to his heart as moderate to severe.

I stood next to my husband's bed as he was drugged for emergency stint surgery, and I was allowed to kiss only his forehead. The realities of what this meant hit me—dead heart tissue, like dead brain tissue and dead eye tissue, never comes back. With as much dead tissue as he had, my dream of us growing old together was gone. It was imperative I understand that my husband was going to die a young man. He was thirty-five years old and had no family history of heart disease and no risk factors for heart disease—but he was going to die. Wrapping my mind around that, I knew we were being blessed with precious time. It would be time filled with happiness. We would have laughter and good memories. I asked the doctor, "So are you saying we have like ten years?" hoping he would say, *Oh no, much more than that.* Instead, he patted my arm and said, "Good, be positive!" Somehow that didn't feel comforting.

The kids were now three and six, and I started practicing what I would say to them. I had to keep reminding myself that this was not about me—it was about them. As I did so, that line became another mantra. My children were not to be burdened with the full emotion of the situation. I would not rob them of the joyful innocence of childhood. *It was not about me.* I needed to be calm as I explained to my children that Daddy had a problem with his heart—the thing that is like your batteries—and that we would need to be very gentle with him when he came home. "Oh, like the bus!" Nathaniel said, making a splat motion with his hands as he remembered the bus accident. Ailsa danced around blowing kisses.

"Yes, like that," I said, referring to the bus accident, "but this time his ouchies are on the inside."

Nathaniel suddenly looked at me grimly, and I could sense his eyes connecting with a piece of knowledge that was almost too great for him to confront. "My toys don't work without batteries," he quietly said.

I could have lied to him. I could have told him that the doctors would get a new battery and that, just like his toys, his daddy's "battery" would be easily fixed. Bringing him into my arms, hoping my soul could say what my mouth couldn't, I said, "That is right." From within the vantage point of my arms, he looked at his sister, who was still dancing around the room, enjoying the chance to perform for me and my mother. I don't know how much he really understood. I like to think that he understood that his little sister didn't need to understand about hearts and batteries. My nickname for Nathaniel had always been Little Man. That day it fit him for more than the reasons he'd originally received it, like being the biggest baby in the nursery—the only baby who had a six-pack.

Immediately after that, I found out I was pregnant. If this baby was going to go full-term, I prayed that it would have memories of its dad. We had changed hospitals to be with the best in a multistate area. They had confirmed the original prognosis. This time Nathan wasn't drugged—he heard it all. He responded with total silence. It must have been hideous for him to hear—to be so young, so healthy, and to realize that there was really nothing that could be done. He squeezed my hand while I mentally repeated my new mantra: "This isn't about me. This is about him, and about Nathaniel and Ailsa."

We had what we jokingly called "old people problems"—lots of medicine, numerous doctor appointments, talks about insurance . . . and more tests . . . were now upon us. We had known old age would eventually come, but suddenly it was here! Nathan is a man of action. The knowledge that he would be leaving us a lot sooner than planned simply increased that trait. We didn't like to talk about what was coming, but he would remind me where all the documents were. We agreed that I would continue to work so we could have some insurance, but what really worried him was Nathaniel and Ailsa not having a dad. Others assured me that I would remarry, but you can guess how helpful that was! I had my Prince Charming—I didn't want a replacement! We considered our marriage to be eternal. His death would not change that—he would forever be my best friend, my lover, and my hubby. I didn't tell him just yet that I was pregnant. I didn't tell anyone. My pregnancy history was stark, and there was enough of death looming over us.

Another round of tests came, this time to determine how much of the stunned heart tissue had since died during the month after the heart attack. I noticed the furrowed eyebrows of the technician and the let's-just-look-at-this-again face. Reminding myself that the emotional response of a freaked-out wife was not what Nathan needed, I silently repeated my mantra: "It is not about me. It is about him, the kids." Our room filled with doctors—never a good sign. With all those experts crowded into our room, the test results must have been very bad. Picking his words very carefully, the doctor slowly said, "You do not have dead heart tissue."

Silence. We stared at the doctor. We were both confused. They had pounded into us the reality of the dead heart tissue. What did this new information mean? Had both hospitals and numerous tests been wrong? I repeated, "He didn't have dead heart tissue?"

The doctor replied directly but kindly, "He *did*, but he doesn't now."

Nathan grabbed my hands and we both said amen, whispered like a prayer. The doctor smiled and nodded his head. A miracle had happened. No medical procedure, drugs, or holistic approaches could have accomplished this. The doctors were there not to give us bad news, but to witness a miracle. As we walked out, the whole office was quietly congratulating us. It was a miracle.

We felt keenly aware that people in other rooms were not getting such good news, and we wondered: Why we were given this when others weren't? We passed through a waiting room full of worried faces with furrowed brows and knew we had been given a new beginning. I felt a little guilty holding my hubby's hand, patting my stomach. Perhaps this pregnancy that God wanted so much would be a baby that I could hold in my arms just eight months from now. It was then that I told my hubby that we were pregnant for the tenth time.

Good news or bad, it always comes down to this. Hotness—surviving life with graciousness and courage, and finding and savoring the joy (especially if there are others who need to lean on your strength)—is about knowing what you can control: *your* response and *your*self. And a huge part of that is letting go once you know you can't control something. The pressure will always be there, whether in big doses or small. You can let it pulverize you—or turn you into a diamond.

Hotness Challenge

If you're like most of the rest of humanity, the load you carry is a whole lot heavier than it needs to be! I'm not talking your arms, thighs, or stomach. I'm talking your mental and emotional load—a load that generally FAR EXCEEDS any love that is clinging to your midsection.

And here's the worst of it: Most of that load is completely unnecessary. It's clinging to you like white on rice, but chances are good that it's not doing you any favors. In fact, chances are good that it's weighing you down in some really unfortunate ways.

That's the bad news. Here's the good news: *You can let it go.* That's right. You can choose to let go of the stuff that is holding you back, weighing you down, making your journey through life more difficult than it needs to be.

Sound great? It is! And here's one way you can make that happen:

1. Notebook in hand, find a place that is warm, comfy, quiet, and free from distractions. You need to be able to concentrate on the important exercise you're about to do.

2. You're going to make two lists. Let's focus on the first one now. Think about the things that are most important in your life—the best in your life, the people and things that give you hope, that help you choose to be the very best you can be. Don't overthink this; for most, it will be a relatively short list. It might include your family, your God, your faith, your home, your best friends, your ability to read or play a musical instrument . . . you get the idea. Jot down the things that bring you real joy, the things you want in your life forever.

3. On a fresh page, start your second list. This one might take more time; in fact, you might have to do it in a few different sessions. On this list, write the things you're carrying around that you want to get rid of. The burdens. The hurt. The pain from an episode that still gnaws at you two decades later. All those things that, when it comes right down to it, you can really do without—would be *much* happier without—but figured you *had* to keep lugging around. Ugly, aren't they? These items are keeping you from being the hottest you can be, and it's time to let go.

4. Now for some powerful imagery. Imagine a box. You decide how big it is, but it needs to hold all that stuff you want to let go of. Put the box down right in the middle of your mind, and start filling it up. One at a time, let go of the things you don't want to carry around anymore. Put each one in the box. Keep going until you're done. If you have to come back to it tomorrow, that's okay.

5. Look up from your work. Just a short distance away stands your God. As you gaze into His eyes, you understand that He is willing to take your box—He is willing to take from you every hurt, every burden, every pain. Carry your box over to Him and put it at His feet.

6. With all your heart, thank Him for taking those things you let go of. Walk away with gratitude and hope, having chosen freedom.

7. With your pain in the past, open your eyes and read over the first list you made—the list of things most important in your life.

8. Choose just one thing on that list and make a plan for how you will focus more intently on that one thing for the next week.

This is an exercise that will probably need to be repeated periodically in your life. Take a few minutes now to enjoy the feeling of relief you experienced when you placed that box at the feet of someone who was willing to take it from you. Breathe deeply and relish the feeling of being free from those burdens. Jot down some reflections on how this exercise has helped increase your hotness.

Never forget that this experience is available to you anytime you need it—and always remember how much hotter you are when you're focused on what's most important in your life!

Chapter Twelve

IT ALL COMES DOWN TO YOUR PERSPECTIVE
CONNECTING TO WHAT MATTERS IN LIFE

L IFE HAS A WAY of testing a person's patience and faith. All of us are given trials to help us grow, and in our case the trials ended in two beautiful children and a happy, healthy father/hubby. Sometimes our trials don't have the happy ending we are hoping for. At times like those it is important to look past what we consider earthly miracles and to know that our loving Heavenly Father also blesses us with celestial miracles.

The numerous miscarriages and the bicycle accident of my youth all combined to make pregnancy hard on me. When I was pregnant with Nathaniel I remember thinking that the way I felt was not normal, but what could I do? I was the sole support of my family, and I was hardly in a position to pamper myself. I would just walk it off. And that is what I tried to do.

By the time Nathaniel was about fifteen months old—ironically, just as he was starting to walk—I realized that the ferocious pain I felt when walking, regardless of its cause, was not going away. I told myself, "Okay, little girl"—a pet name I call myself—"you're gimpy. So what? Get a good attitude."

Walking became more and more painful. I tried so hard to hide the pain that all anyone saw was a slight limp. It was almost impossible for me to lift my son, who seemed to weigh as much as a college linebacker. I decided that if he would just start to walk, my problems would be over.

That just showed what I *didn't* know about toddlers once they start to walk. He seemed to go from his first staggering steps to a full-on run in no time. I quickly discovered that running didn't work for me either—my leg wanted to drag behind, and my "run" was anything but graceful. But I had no choice—I had to run after him as he explored streets, lakes, and anything but the playground. Fences around playgrounds should be the law.

When I became pregnant with Ailsa, the physical therapist told me to stay down. When I asked her if she had kids, she said no. Perhaps it was not kind of me, but I told her that someday when she had a two-and-a-half-year-old boy to remember that she told me to stay down and rest. My husband was doing an internship in Washington, DC, living there with some dear friends. I was on my own, and I was expected to stay down? Sure. That would work! I would just let the child run loose! Luckily my church family came to my aid, organizing play dates and taking me to medical appointments.

In September 2008, three months pregnant with my third child, I was placed on bed rest—that's what we called it. Most pregnant women are put on bed rest to prevent the threat of early labor, but my bed rest was due to what we now knew to be my SI joint and back issues. I was in severe pain—real, blinding pain—twenty-four hours a day, seven days a week. It never let up; toward the end I was passing out from pain. There was no medication I could have; my only treatment was from my physical therapist, Damon Aguirre. As I walked, my nerves would spasm, sending pain through the entire left side of my body. I described it like a knife in my hip. (Granted, I have never been stabbed. But I did cut a very small piece of my fingertip off once—this hurt worse.)

I was to use a cane. They are great for gentleman in old movies— very debonair. My mother, who has MS, has canes with character—

some are made from tree roots. Some people carve faces in theirs; once I saw a man with flames painted on his. Okay, so some canes are cool. But at thirty-five, I was embarrassed to have one. I *was* glad for the help it gave me, and soon I learned where to hide it when sitting so I only looked tragic when walking. I sat a lot. But when the nerves went off I was glad to have it so I didn't fall. Soon I had two canes— two are better than one from a medical perspective—but to me it was impossible to hide that I was holding on for dear life with each step. Determined to stay out of a wheelchair, I was moved to a walker.

Walkers are not as glamorous as you may first think. Sure, you always have a built-in chair with you, but if you encounter even the slightest downgrade, like those found on regular old sidewalks, the walker picks up speed. I just knew the walker would eventually pick up enough speed that it would drag me behind it. Horrific. Our church family—who had served us through the bus accident with meals and play dates, and through the heart attack with more meals and longer play dates—dedicated countless hours of service and prayers to us. By Christmas I was in a wheelchair.

I may have been in a wheelchair, but my children—who were only four and seven—were absolute troopers. They learned to make their own peanut butter sandwiches. Nathaniel once got sent off to afternoon kindergarten without me reminding him to eat. He came home from school hungry, but before getting himself something, he brought me a leftover yam from the fridge, thinking of me before himself. The kids made do, assuming tasks that were once mine. I had to watch, terrified, as four-year-old Ailsa struggled up the stairs with her basket of laundry. As I was mostly stationary, the children often found me in bed, and cuddled with my tummy as much as they did with me. Ailsa would lift up my shirt and place her head on the baby, giving her kisses and talking about all the fun things they would do.

Our tenth pregnancy was five months along when we found out we were having a girl! We picked the name Katelynn, meaning "pure," and a middle name of Faith. The physical suffering seemed worth it; I was going to hold a baby. The day after Christmas I went in for what I thought was a routine ultrasound. Actually, it was an extra that had been ordered for me; because of my history, they were being cautious. I wasn't worried; my tummy was growing, and I felt Katelynn kicking.

At the doctor's office, a woman in the waiting room asked how long I'd been on bed rest. I told her. She was stunned and replied, "Oh, I just couldn't do that! I'm much too valuable to my family!" *Evidently I'm not!* I laughed inside. You never know how much you can adapt until you have to.

The last trimester was to be hell. The pain seemed beyond what I could bear, but it wasn't just physical pain. Our sweet Katelynn Faith had some issues. They told us it looked like it might be trisomy 18, a condition they told me was "incompatible with life." In other words, nothing could be done. I could induce labor now instead of drawing out what would eventually happen anyway—her death. Why put me through more physical and emotional suffering when my ability to be fully mobile after pregnancy was already in question?

There had been some concerns with Ailsa early on, and one doctor had suggested that I terminate my pregnancy with her. So we had been down this road before, and Ailsa was a perfectly healthy child. Nathan and I just looked at each other. Neither one of us considered inducing labor. We knew that Katelynn was ours and that she was a miracle. Nathan was alive. We had seen miracles; we were confident that we would see another. And we did.

We choose to do an amniocentesis. I couldn't go home and tell Nathaniel and Ailsa that their sister was only going to live a short time if that wasn't a complete certainty. After all, I had said as much after their dad's heart attack and he had been healed. I could start to lose credibility with my kids if I told them someone was dying every few months!

Katelynn Faith didn't have trisomy 18. Instead she had very rare issues that the doctors didn't know much about. She had inherited a strain of my chromosomal anomaly that had caused the miscarriages and possibly some of my structural issues. You know the X-men in the movies? They were genetic mutants, and so was I! Unfortunately, though, I didn't get any cool superhero power that lets me repeatedly save the world. In our hopes, we knew that Katelynn's differences had made her special and she would be given every opportunity to find her way in life.

The one thing that we did know about Katelynn was that she had a heart condition that was very fixable. The cardiologist was not worried—he assured us that this kind of condition was successfully repaired all the time. The only other organs that were slightly compromised were her kidneys. Other than that, things were pretty much a mystery. Only two other babies were known to have Katelynn's same chromosomal issues, and they had both been aborted. No matter, we thought—not all children are tested *in utero*, and we were sure that other people were walking around with her same chromosomal pattern, living normal lives.

Katelynn Faith was born April 1, 2009. A team of twenty-one people attended her birth. There was a terrifying moment when she wasn't breathing, and I came close to hysteria waiting to be told she was okay. After the doctors finished evaluating her, a process that took many hours, I was wheeled in to see my brown-haired little girl. She looked just like me, complete with the sturdy shoulders of my dad's side. She had the Maughan family build. They were strong people, miners in England and laborers in America who had immigrated to worship God, only to be attacked by mobs. The ancestor from whom our large family descended had pushed a handcart west and had been caught in an early winter; hundreds of those with him had died.

Katelynn came from strong people. She was strong. She squeezed my finger and as I held her, she looked at me. I was her mom. I had a connection to her stronger than I had with either of my other two, perhaps because I had suffered so much physically to get her here. Being taken from her bedside was agony, and when I was discharged from the hospital and she remained behind, being so far from my baby was the hardest thing in my life to that point.

During her time in the hospital she seemed to be in such a cold, sterile environment filled with monitors and tubes. The nurse said to me, "There is something special about Katelynn." She was right. I didn't want to see it, but Katelynn was very special. She didn't stare at lights; she didn't fight the daily blood tests; she was attentive to people, giving direct eye contact. She looked right at you, right into your soul. Every day at two a friend would pick me up at my home; because of my nerve issues I was still in a wheelchair and couldn't drive. I would be at Katelynn's bed by three. Nathan would come after work, and we would be with her until they kicked us out at seven thirty for rounds and shift change. Katelynn came to anticipate my arrival. Her heart rate would go up and then go down as I came to bed number 17, her place in Primary Children's NICU. She knew I was her mom.

One day I was given some bad news. Thanking the doctors for their professionalism, I went back to connecting with my baby girl. She looked at me, and she looked at them—she was always looking at someone. The social worker came and asked why I hadn't cried. They were concerned that I didn't get it—I was simply too happy . . . too cheerful . . . too *not* sad. The nurses who were with Katelynn and me laughed off the others' concerns that I just didn't get it. Those who knew me and Katelynn knew what I was doing. I'd made a decision, very deliberately, that I was going to give Katelynn my best. Because I am her mom, I wouldn't break down in a slobbery mess in front of her any more than I would in front of her brother and sister.

Every day I got dressed up as nicely as I could and did my makeup. I stole a line from my mom, who says she gets dressed up because she wants to look worth saving! Being in a wheelchair as I headed to visit my baby in the NICU was tragic enough—I didn't need to look like a mess on top of it all. Every day I did my Vanity Prayers, and I saw myself being awesome. No, I didn't wake up feeling that way; every day my first conscious thought at waking up was the pain. It was there all the time, even in my sleep, but it was so much worse as I became conscious each morning, trying to suck me into its bitter mood. I had to create the vision of being awesome.

Sitting on my bedside looking at my wheelchair every morning, I had an open conversation with God. I would look at what was before me that day. Every task, each moment demanded more than I had. If I had to put a percentage on what I thought I could do physically, emotionally, or spiritually, that percentage was always below 10 percent. Just getting ready was so hard, so draining. I told God that that the other 90 percent—sometimes 98 percent—was on Him. I had to be amazing. I had to awesome. I had to be beyond my best for the many who were looking to my attitude to see if they could get through this. I would not let them down because I was their mom.

Nathaniel and Ailsa spent more time with me in the day than anyone else. Katelynn had nurses who loved her tenderly, but I was still her mom; we had shared a heartbeat. I was the constant and I had to be consistently beyond what I could be. God gave me that strength. I say this to glorify Him, not me—I was able to do my best each day with the highest of hopes because of the strength He gave me. I know that many prayers were given in our behalf.

I felt depleted by having my three children in two separate places, by the physical pain that mounted during pregnancy and did not go away after childbirth, and by the fact there was so much of the unknown, so much over which I didn't have control. But I *did* have control over my attitude.

One day I wheeled myself through the hospital lobby, trying to pump myself up but failing miserably. My morning Vanity Prayers had been depleted from the needs of my children and—as if the situation I was facing wasn't enough—from extended family drama. Arriving at the hospital I felt small and unable to do what was needed of me. I reminded myself that I had strength greater than what I thought I had. Being open to that strength sounds so easy, doesn't it? We get so determined to stay in our grumpy bear mood, justifying why we should get to stay exactly as we are: grumpy, miserable, and stuck. That's fun, isn't it? Whatever the situation, you can slump in defeat or stand in assurance of the strength that will come. And you can start by smiling.

That's what I did that day. Well, I didn't stand, but I smiled as I wheeled my chair through the hospital lobby. The front desk attendant smiled at me. A woman stood in my path, smiling as I approached; she told me she had noticed before that I was always smiling. Gesturing to a young man, she asked if I would talk to her son and tell him how I chose to be happy in a chair.

It was like the camera of my life was in clear focus. The young man before me was very physically limited. He didn't have use of his hands; they were turned in and could barely reach the controls on his chair. In contrast, my arms were in the best shape they had been in years, toned from the canes and the walker and now the chair. I could wheel myself wherever there was a ramp. His condition, I presumed, had existed since birth; mine had existed for only a few months. I felt guilty at the childhood I had of running through chest-high grasses, climbing trees, building forts, jumping, and working. My body had let me work hard alongside my brothers and my father, building, making an earning. The boy in this chair had so much less than I had. Even if I was forever limited, my worst was better than his best. The smile I wore had drawn us together; his mother wanted me to give advice to him. What could I say?

God gave me the answer. I told him about facing the hard things in life with a good attitude, that some of us wore our pain on the outside but we all had pain, difficulty, and loss. We didn't know by looking at another person what his or her story was. I told him that he would inspire all he met as he faced his challenges and chose to face them well. I told him that he would find joy, even when it was hard. He could serve others, have an impact, and his own difficulties would be easier to bear. I was thinking of my own worst challenge as I spoke—of my worries for Katelynn.

Had I not been smiling that day, a mother and son would have seen one more rain cloud wheeling herself around. How many of us are rain clouds? Is it really that hard to smile, to choose to be a light—to amplify the rays of good instead of the gloom and doom we all feel? "Happy" people are people who have chosen to focus on the good even when life is really poopy at times.

For Mother's Day I announced to the other moms that we would be having a special party. I arranged to have a TV brought in, and we watched *Bride and Prejudice: Bollywood Meets Jane Austen*, a great colorful movie with a cheese factor that makes you want to dance along. We held our babies, which in my case involved a team of people to move her into my arms. And we celebrated something normal—that was also the day that my children were able, under special arrangements, to get to meet Katelynn. It was a perfect day. All of us were together. It was our last Mother's Day as a family.

Katelynn was going to have heart surgery. It was her only option if she was to go forward. She ended up having two surgeries in thirty-six hours because the first one didn't go well. There was a long wait, and an even longer night where I prayed, pleading for my baby girl. I asked God, who had given me so much, to give me this too. That night, May 17, she looked me in the eye, and we communicated. I could see in her eyes that she was tired. She wanted to rest. I told her that I couldn't be without her.

She held on that night for me, until I was ready to do what Katelynn needed me to do: face her death. On May 24, 2009, Katelynn returned to her Father in Heaven. I was holding her in my arms as she went; my husband was holding me in his arms.

Katelynn lived for fifty-four precious days. I will share her story, her life, her death, and all of what she taught us in a book I have titled *More Laughter Than Tears*. This book, however, has a different purpose. It is to teach that regardless of where you come from, regardless of what you experience, you have the power to decide your own potential and attitude. You do it through controlling what you choose to think about and what you do with the time in your life. I share a small piece of Katelynn with you now because of one of the most profound things she taught us.

She looked everyone in the eye. She was here to learn, to soak up the amazing people around her. When I held her in my arms, Katelynn would look directly at anyone who walked within gazing distance. This is why the nurses called her special. She *was* special—more special than I would have liked her to be, because she was apparently too pure to remain on earth. She looked at us as I know God looks at us—with interest, love, and straight into our soul.

The irony is that for years I had been teaching women to look in the mirror and to love themselves—to look right into their soul, to look into their subconscious mind and to say nice things to affirm what is right, not what is wrong. Katelynn did that. She could express everything she needed in her fifty-four days of life without the ability to cry or laugh—she did it all with her eyes. More than four hundred people came to her funeral. In the years since her death people mention her to us and tell us about the impact she had on their lives. That impact—the lessons she taught everyone she touched—is still being felt. She was one person who saw.

I don't think that Katelynn's eternal potential is any greater than anyone else's. I think her life purpose was short, but she is still learning, loving, and teaching. She is still teaching me. I joke that out of my three children, Katelynn is the most demanding of my time and talents. It is because of her that I stepped out of living my life safely into what was possible. It is because I want her to look in on her mom choosing to be happy, productive, and powerful with the time I have.

Look at yourself. Strip away your excuses, your fears, your cannots. You have more time and ability to do than did my daughter Katelynn and the many other babies who die before they really begin to live. You have a purpose. You have abilities—some you know about and some that are still untapped. Yet your self-doubt, anger, and poopy talk hold you back from the joy you can have.

Katelynn had impact because she knew who she was. She knew why she was here and she lived her life really connecting with others. Live like she did. Find out why you are here by daily connecting—not as a result of the gurus of mentoring, though they can be a tool, but as a result of the ultimate course of knowing who you are and why you are here. Those answers will be given to you by the source of truth—God. You will find God looking into His most amazing creation—you. Look into your eyes and stop beating up what you see. Be open to the hotness inside of you!

I was a shy, insecure, talentless, and emotionally rung-out child. Now I'm a mother, a wife—successful, happy, and all the other adjectives you want to add on. I'm not talking about rags to riches, but about sad to happy. From poopy to hotness. I have done great things not because I set out to do them but because I didn't quit.

Life is hard; none of us can predict what will happen. The only thing we have control over is our attitude and what we teach our children. We will all have situations that will leave us reeling. We can fall into bitterness or we can decide to teach another message. We are a product of what we focus on.

The light, the hotness, is with you. The best way to make it grow is to feed it. Which will you feed? The darkness or the light? When you feed the light, you not only help yourself but spark the light in others as well. Be like Katelynn—be the light. Be the connection to all things good and pure. It is your decision.

Choose.

Hotness Challenge

As much as we try to look on the bright side, here's the bitter truth: Sometimes really crummy things happen in life. In this chapter I shared with you the events leading up to Katelynn Faith's life. And her death.

When I think of all the things I would have chosen on my journey, her death is sure not one of them. Yes, I learned some life-changing lessons. I came out of the experience stronger, more sure of myself, more determined to love and cherish the people I still had on this earth. But there's no getting around it: Had I been able to choose, I would have wished for her a long, happy, and healthy life. I would have wished for myself in the bargain the chance to gather her into my arms and coach her through that long, happy, and healthy life.

I didn't share my experience with you so you would feel sorry for me. I shared my experience with you so you could see that it's possible to come out of something really horrific *still* connected to the things that really matter in your life. That even if you have significant problems (and most of us do at one time or another), you can still find the good. That even when despair claws at you relentlessly, you can still feel gratitude.

You can be a light—to yourself and others—even in the worst of circumstances. Here's how:

1. No matter what is going on in your life, make the decision to give your very best to those you love. When all is said and done, those people are the things that matter most in your life. Remember my mantra from the last chapter? *This isn't about me—this is about them.* At least once each day, determine one thing you can do for one of the people who matter most in your life. Then do it.

2. Start a gratitude or happiness journal. I did one of these in my twenties to help me start healing. Get an inexpensive journal. Then, every night after your Vanity Prayers, write down at least one thing for which you are grateful. *No fair repeating!* Make each entry unique. Afraid you'll run out of things to write? Don't worry. None of us ever could.

At the end of a week, assess your progress. Are you feeling happier? More grateful? Hotter? The longer you do this exercise, the more joy and contentment you will radiate. The more joy and contentment you radiate, the more others will want to be around you. Because you'll be *hot*!

Chapter Thirteen

~

NOW YOU KNOW WHAT DOESN'T MATTER
LETTING GO TO HONOR YOU

CINDERELLA was the best of women. Her character was above question; she was so kind even little animals liked her. She was patient with those who were cruel to her. When her prince swooped her away to the castle and she rode off to her happily ever after, she showed her truly good heart. Because of this she *deserved* her happily ever after with her prince.

But let's get real. Life isn't a fairy tale. Things are a little harder to tie up so nicely. Life is hard. People hurt us. We want to have things resolved. We don't often get those tidy, happy endings. From the outside, it looks like Cinderella got everything she could ever want. Why? If we believe Cinderella to be as good, kind, and patient as she is portrayed to be, she had to learn to focus on the best of her life, not the worst. She got the good life had to offer because she had hope. She had hope in herself and she had hope for others.

Never in any of the versions I have seen or read of the classic fairy tale did those who wronged Cinderella apologize to her. But she had hope for others, so she forgave them anyway, even if they didn't ask for forgiveness. She didn't hold on to the pain. She let it go. She didn't ride off into the sunset with her prince being bitter about the past and bringing every wrong along with them on the white horse. She left that bitterness and those wrongs where they belonged—behind her. She didn't even think about letting them impact her current happiness.

How do we follow Cinderella's example? Or, an even deeper question, how do we choose to be our best self? How do we become what God wants us to be? There is not a moment that everything is perfect, that everything goes together just right and we ride away from our problems. It's only after we decide to leave the pain in the past that we can see clearly. We have to forgive first! And we can't wait for someone to apologize before we forgive, because seldom do people apologize.

I shared with you that my grandmother said some poopy things to me. She shouldn't have said those kinds of things. My grandparents should have looked at me through eyes of hope for my future. They owed me an apology. Instead, they insisted on pointing out my failings at every opportunity, even when I was an adult. *My* turning point in our relationship came when I was almost twenty-three— when I'd returned from serving a mission for my church and I had a 4.0 grade-point average in college. My work was going great; I was the most-requested interpreter for the deaf at the Washington, DC, children's hospital, and the young man I was dating had a question he wanted to ask me when I returned from a family trip. He was a great man, the kind of guy that parents or grandparents would want. It seemed that my happily ever after was about to start!

But before I could find happily ever after, there was this family trip. I joined my sister and cousins on a history tour of my grandfather's childhood home in Nebraska. My grandparents were showing us where he grew up, the church he attended, the school he went to, and the areas in which he worked and played; we also got to hear stories about him shared by those he knew. What an experience! I could almost see him as a young man.

Then things went all wrong. I said something—I don't even remember what—but apparently it was not the right thing to say. My grandfather began yelling at me. I remember it like it was yesterday. I was sitting in the back of the van. My cousins were looking at me awkwardly. And my grandfather—the one whose life we had been studying and *honoring*—was painting me out to be everything wrong with the world. He saw weakness in me, and he shared that weakness with everyone there. I was beyond humiliated. But just as the darkness of self-doubt was beginning to blacken what had seemed the perfect future, I had an epiphany: *I wasn't the one with the problem!*

True, the Ten Commandments insist that we honor our father and mother—and I had always believed this meant I should also honor my grandparents. But maybe I was going about it all wrong. And now I wondered: did *honor* mean to blindly accept whatever my parents or grandparents handed out? I *had* brought honor to my family by my good life; my life choices had been in line with what God had asked that I do. I was a good person. Yet here I was being yelled at by a person I was supposed to honor, a list of my faults being recited at top decibel as the mile markers whizzed by.

I started recalling all the unkind things my grandparents had ever said to me. Even though I graduated high school with honors, I almost flunked out of college during my sophomore year because I was working full-time, going to school full-time, and battling an illness. Despite those challenges, I was held up as an utter disappointment. The fact that I had been diagnosed with a serious case of Epstein Barr didn't matter. I knew I had failed and I believed I was stupid. This was emphasized by the fact that I was the only grandchild who had not received any financial help from our grandparents, even though they had promised it. Because of that, I had to work, but that didn't matter either. I finally left school to earn money, and my grandparents were then deeply ashamed that I made that choice. They wrote me a letter telling me so. After working for a time and spending some time in Alaska, I served a mission for my church before returning to school.

After what they perceived as my near dropout, my grandparents promised that when I got a 4.0 they would help me with my schooling. But now that I had the required grade-point average, they said I "wasn't worth the investment," that "the funds were better used on others." I was devastated by those words. And sitting in the van that day, I realized that only my failures were going to be remembered. Only the shame was recited. No allowance was made for the positive things I had done. The 4.0 wasn't enough. It wasn't even mentioned. Nothing I could ever do could redeem me in their eyes.

If I was working to prove to them that I was worthy of respect, love, or even kind words, my motives were wrong. I had to honor myself. I had to be motivated not by selfishness, not by pride, not by glory, and not to gain validation and praise from others. I had to look at what really motivated me.

Letting my grandparents define my worth, my potential, and my purpose was my choice. As long as I was seeking their approval, I couldn't be working for my own approval. I was not bringing honor to others by doing good only to please them. I was just a rat in a cage, scurrying to do the tricks assigned to me. I had to honor my purpose—I needed to do what was right simply because it was the right action: to first honor myself.

The year before I sat in the back of the van listening to my grandfather's blistering diatribe, I had spent a significant chunk of my life serving and giving to others—teaching them to pray, teaching them to read the scriptures, teaching them about the Atonement of Jesus Christ. I had shared with others the ultimate hope for each of us—that in our failings and shame of our own making, or the hurt and shame thrust on us, there was a way to the light of hope. It was an amazing experience. The kind of service, sharing, and learning I did brought me a deeper sense of God's love. It was one of the most profound experiences of my life. I learned that sacrifice puts you in a better position to be blessed—that when we trust God, He holds us.

In that van in Nebraska, I was reminded of what God had already told me at fifteen. I had to decide then and there what I meant to do with that knowledge. At fifteen, I had learned then that a funny name or failures were only events—that what mattered was what I did about those events. What I allowed to define me today was what I did today. I needed to remember in that moment, and always, that no one else can define you; no one else can decide your worth.

I emerged from that van a different woman. I mulled over the lessons, seeing that I would never ride off into my happily ever after if I didn't learn then and there to honor myself. And that was the key to honoring my grandparents and anyone else I loved (despite how they saw me). And I knew instinctively that I needed to let go of all the hurt and wrong that had been done to me, and all the wrong-headed motivations that had been driving me. Because holding on to those wrongs would taint my future.

I might get the prince, but what happily ever after would it be if I spent the nights walking the halls of the castle wringing my hands and asking if others approved? I had to let it go. I had to forgive. They couldn't see me or love me as I wanted, and that had to be okay. That they seemed to love others more was not the point. I had been seeking approval from those who were not apt to be pleased with what I did—or even pleased with me. It was my failing for expecting them to be what I wanted them to be. Ruminating over the pain didn't honor the purpose of my life or the day!

Forgiving those who have hurt you is easier in some cases than others. The less you care about the person, the easier it is to forgive and to let it go. Deeper pain may require some spiritual therapy. Those we love most are the hardest to forgive because we EXPECT so much from them. Let go of the expectation; free them to be what they are. Yes, it is easier to say than do, but it's a process—and an extremely worthwhile one.

Using my Vanity Prayer time to focus on what I want for the day helps me focus on growth and honor instead of licking my wounds.

The Bible gives great advice: ask God for help to forgive and pray for the person who has wronged you. That advice works because when we forgive, we start to release people from what *we* want and start to give them what God would want for them. Remove your judgment and love them without your judgment getting in the way. It is not our business to fix others. Our business is to assess our own growth. As I focused on me, getting motivated to do what was honoring my purpose, I began to feel peace feeding my soul a little more each day.

When we seek for validation from others we are disappointed—and often devastated—when we don't receive it. Instead of losing trust in others, we tend to lose trust in ourselves. Being human, others will disappoint us. Giving trust when others have not earned it will lead us to being hurt and bitter if we don't check our own motives. The responsibility to make us happy or whole is not for others to bear. We are happy when we choose to honor what is right for ourselves and give others freedom and forgiveness. When we do this, we see life differently and can honor others freely without expecting anything in return. But this is the important thing to remember: you can give to others only what you first give yourself.

At the time, there was another consequence to learning this truth about myself and honoring my future. I did not want to choose paths or people in life simply because they validated my worth. This played out painfully at first, as is often the case with daring to change. When I got home, the young man I was dating took me out for a lovely evening; in the moonlight, he got down on one knee and asked me a very important question. He started by saying, "You are amazing." What young lady doesn't what to hear that from a great guy? He listed the qualities of mine that he admired. Then he said, "I think you are the best that has come along." And then he said something about marriage. I didn't really hear him. And he kept talking, but I don't remember exactly what came after that. Why? My mind was stuck on the fact that he thought I was the best that had come along!

That was not the declaration of love I'd been anticipating. I was hearing a good man who admired a girl—but didn't love her—asking her to marry him. My value was all in his mind, not his heart. I was being asked to marry him not because he loved me but for what I had accomplished "on paper." Besides that, I was the best that "had come along." He was *settling* for me.

I knew that would leave me forever worried about pleasing him—for the wrong reasons—and my motivations could again be compromised. I told him that he needed to know he loved me and that he had two weeks to decide. I would say yes if he knew that he did. And then came the part of the fairy tale they never show. I went into the kitchen, leaned against the fridge, collapsed to the floor, and cried until I had no tears left. I loved him. He didn't love me enough. The next morning my sister asked with giddy delight how things had gone. I told her, and the tears came again. He didn't love me enough. I had to say it out loud, and it hurt.

At that point, things got very emotional. My sister said, "Leta, your prince isn't going to come and swoop you up onto a white horse!" I told her that until he did, I would remain single. I disappointed her; I was a silly romantic. She took my hands, looked deep into my eyes, and asked, "How many options do you really have?" (Doesn't life test your resolve to change?!)

The two-week deadline came. He sounded like he was trying to talk himself into loving me. I shook his hand and welcomed him to being my friend. In friend mode I prayed for him to find the right woman. I prayed to honor myself that I wouldn't let the love I felt for him send him mixed signals. We maintained the friendship, demonstrating the good character we both had. It was awkward at times, but I knew that things were as they should be. I released both of us to find our real amazing happily ever after instead of being together just because it was a good fit. Didn't he deserve to start his marriage deeply in awe of—and in love with—his bride? Didn't I deserve the same from my groom?

Leta Greene

Letting him go and forgiving him was easy with the perspective that I was bringing honor to him and to me. As if on cue in a dramatic stage production, the first man I actually wanted to marry because in my heart I knew he loved me came on the scene next and professed his love in storybook perfection. Just looking at him tingled my toes. We had a dramatic romantic relationship of poetry and late-night talks that felt they could never end. But as much as I felt for him, my mind knew we were wrong. I wanted my mind and heart to agree. He left. I cried.

Six months later at a church dance a young man came in, asked me to dance, and the rest is history. I was twenty-four when I became Mrs. Greene. We rode off into the sunset to begin our happily ever after. He loved me enough to make choices before we ever met that honored him and honored his purpose—and the person he was when I met him fit my list. His goals and focus were in line with what I wanted. He loved me enough that when he got down on his knee and asked me to be his wife he promised to honor me. He told me he loved God and that God would always be first. He loved me enough that we were married in God's house and made promises to each other that we would love and honor each other forever.

Each night we are not apart he takes me by the hand and we pray together. Love is choosing to start again—to put aside the hurt and to start each day determined to honor what is right and best for yourself, for those who depend on you, and for your God. When you are married to someone who is focused on the same thing, you enhance each other and your individual efforts are magnified—you are one. Don't give your happiness to those who are not going to love you enough to cherish that trust.

Events in life don't always go as planned, but if you depend on God you can get through those bumps, hits, disappointments, pains, and losses as long as you focus on character and honor. The fair things don't always happen. In fact, things usually don't happen at all, or don't happen when we think they should. That doesn't mean you can't be happy. Happiness can be had each day by liking yourself and leaving the past to fester on itself. Free yourself from the box of perceptions made by others and focus instead on the things given you by God.

When I was thirty-nine years old, Grandma called me and apologized. The miracle as I saw it was not that she apologized. Yes, that was a real surprise; as far as I know, she has never apologized to anyone—nor did her mother before her. In tears, she asked for my forgiveness. No, that wasn't the miracle. The miracle was that when I looked into my heart, I knew I had forgiven her a long time ago. I had been free during all those years to honor my purpose in life and to choose happiness. I had freed her to do what she needed. She was the victim of her own feelings, and I had not been bound by what she felt or said.

There were other surprises in that conversation. Grandma opened up to me with an honesty I have never witnessed from her. She told me of her mother. She told me she was amazed by me—that she respected me. The words I had craved as a child and young adult now flowed eloquently from her. Had I turned on her with venom in that moment of tenderness, we both would have lost something precious. Now we can work on building trust.

Grandma was ninety-three when she made that phone call, and time is a precious and limited thing. Had I waited to forgive her before until I heard her validation, I would have waited almost forty years without getting what I craved. In extending her forgiveness without a timetable of expectation, I was able to be kind to her when we were around each other. I was able to let her comments slide off, and I was able to leave them there.

Had I chosen to do things in a different way, the anger I could have felt would have built bigger, sturdier walls of resentment, hurt, and justification. It really doesn't matter who makes the mud puddle—it matters who jumps in the mud, who gets covered with the muck, and who builds bricks out of the mud. When we build muddy brick walls to protect ourselves, we close ourselves inside and we starve on our own broken unmet expectations and bitter hearts. If we fill ourselves with a diet of justification about what is owed us, the empty calories block out the ability to choose joy. We are the ones who starve while paying the price—not the person who put the mud there. The one who USES the mud to make bricks dies of a broken, bitter heart.

When we forgive others, we move away from the mud battlefield. Stay out of the mud; it is really stinky. Mud is easy to make. But just because it is easy to make doesn't make it honorable. In fact, honor is not easy; it is created day after day, month after month, over a sustained period of time.

By the way, that man who thought he wanted to marry me? His heart and mind *did* find his queen, and they are living happily ever after as well.

Hotness Challenge

Somewhere along your pathway of life—in fact, in *lots* of places along that pathway—someone will hurt you. Offend you. Say or do something so unimaginably heartless that you can scarcely believe it. Oh, it's rarely premeditated or planned to any degree. While there are definitely a few monsters dotting the planet—and sometimes the people who should love us most end up weaving a lifelong tapestry of monstrous cruelty—most of the time things get said or done in the passion of the moment. And the old "sticks and stones" verse? They had it wrong. Words can inflict the most painful injuries of all. And while broken bones heal, the wounds associated with careless or cruel words can last a lifetime. *If we let them.*

You mean there's a choice?

Listen to what bestselling author Sarah Ban Breathnach had to say: "Today expect something good to happen to you no matter what occurred yesterday. Realize the past no longer holds you captive. It can only continue to hurt you if you hold on to it. Let the past go.

A simply abundant world awaits" (*Simple Abundance: A Daybook of Comfort and Joy* [New York: Grand Central], 2005).

How do you let go?

Forgive.

While forgiveness can be supremely difficult, it is always worth the effort. Why? As renowned Christian author, ethicist, and theologian Lewis B. Smedes put it, "To forgive is to set a prisoner free and discover that the prisoner was you." In his typical positive outlook, humorist and author Mark Twain quipped, "Forgiveness is the fragrance that the violet sheds on the heel that has crushed it."

This Hotness Challenge is truly a *challenge*, because forgiveness is rarely easy. By now, though, you *know* you can do hard things. And forgiveness, while hard, is one of the best things you can do: If you want to move forward with happiness, you must leave the bitterness behind. Forgiveness is the key.

Ready?

1. On a small slip of paper, write down the name of the person you most need to forgive. This probably won't take a lot of thought: Chances are, you live with the hurt that person caused every day of your life. Most likely, it's front and center. So write down the name.

2. Fold the paper in half and slip it into your pocket. Make sure it's there, where you can feel it, every time you put your hand in that pocket. Remember the name—even more than you usually do.

3. Have a good cry. (When I say *have a good cry*, I mean for an hour or two. I don't mean for weeks.) Mourn for your vulnerability at the time you got hurt, and feel real sorrow for the person who hurt you so badly. That's right. *Feel sorrow for the person who hurt you.* Imagine, if you can,

how badly that person must have been hurting to want to strike out at you in that way. Imagine what an empty life that person must have been living. Weep for the time and energy and passion that has been wasted by all your hurt. Then stop crying. Wipe your tears. Blow your nose. Think how *absolutely wonderful* it will feel when you no longer have to cry over this.

4. Pray for the ability to forgive. Pray, because letting go of that kind of hurt and betrayal is blisteringly difficult to do without help. Pray, because you'll need support. In a small notebook, record how your feelings begin to change about the person whose name is on the slip of paper you feel every day in your pocket.

5. If you feel that you need professional support in addition to prayer or other religious support, seek it. Continue to record how you feel—not only about the other person, but about yourself.

There's no time schedule attached to this challenge because forgiveness is not an instant thing. It takes time. It takes effort. It might take years. But how free—and HOT—you will be at the end of the process. So what if the person never apologizes? Be very clear on this: the person you forgive may never find out you've forgiven him or her. But *you know.* In this instance, *you're* the one who benefits. And that's not all: you have the kind of character that extends forgiveness as a gift, never expecting anything in return. And that is one of the hottest qualities of all!

Chapter Fourteen

---------------- ✿ ----------------

WHAT'S *YOUR* DIET?
MOTIVATION AND FOCUSING ON A HOT FUTURE

W E ARE HERE ON EARTH. We are alive, hopefully healthy, and we can be anything we want to be. So, what is your motivation? I love chocolate. I notice every study that says it is good for me. I reject any study that says otherwise. Just having it in my house makes me happy; I don't have to eat it—just knowing it is there is enough. I love it. I love everything about it—the texture, the taste, the melt. Santa puts gourmet dark chocolate in my stocking every year. Santa is awesome.

So, you know how I feel about chocolate. But it's not the main thing I eat. My main diet is made up of green leafy salads, veggies, fruits, water, and milk (because it falls in the same category as chocolate—health nuts, back off). The meat I eat is "happy meat," meaning it was happy during its life instead of being cooped up in a coop. Most of the fish I eat swam free. None of what I eat is covered in chocolate. Oh, except raisins and pomegranates seeds—seriously, you gotta get some!

So why do I eat things that are good for me? Why don't I limit myself to the stuff I really love—chocolate-covered dairy-blissful happiness? I try to eat right because I like how my body feels when I do. I have noticed that if I drink soda my body is tired and my throat is little sore the next morning.

I eat right because I want to be healthy, not because I am trying to be thinner. I have decided that how I look right now is just fine. I am not trying to beat out anyone else as the top hottie. How I am is hot enough.

As a result of the way I eat, I maintain a very consistent weight. When I'm not pregnant, I weigh within twenty pounds of what I did in high school. If I want to be thinner, though diet plays a role, I have to work out. I choose to "exercise" only because I enjoy walking, so I need to do enough physical therapy to keep my body working right.

Those are the things that motivate me.

Motivation is a fascinating thing. What motivates us? Billions are spent every year by people who are trying to buy motivation—to get into shape, to be healthy, to be happy, to be successful. Gurus promise us motivation. I'm called a *motivational speaker*, but I don't really like that title. Why? Because motivation comes from within! We may be motivated temporarily by fear or want, but eventually we will become accustomed to the push and accept that what we are is okay. We lose our willpower for our New Year's resolutions by January 20, and by February 14 we wonder why others don't love us enough to spoil us with a box of chocolates.

Zig Zigler said, "People often say that motivation doesn't last. Well, neither does bathing. That's why we recommend it daily." It's not a moment of clarity that changes us; it is a commitment to the clarity, frequently practiced, that changes us, that motivates us to change.

Motivation is only part of the trick—we can be motivated by fear, thinness, and chocolate only so long. Sure, I wouldn't mind perfect abs that I could post on Pinterest. (Okay, I wouldn't actually ever do that.) We would all like to be perfect—who wouldn't? We all like the idea of it, but we don't do it. We diet and fail, we intend to and don't, and billions of dollars are being made yearly off all of us who are trying to be perfect.

So if motivation is only part of the secret, what's the rest? As Zig Zigler is implying, it's *focus*. When we place our focus on the right thing, we can maintain the activity required to get the result we want. Get a vision of what you can become if what you want to do what is hard. Now work on keeping that vision fresh. Do it today. That is why I start my day with Vanity Prayers. Every day I see that day full of possibility; I plan on being awesome. I tell myself that I can do what the day asks of me. I get dressed for the purpose of the day. I not only look the part, but I tell the world by how I look that I mean to be amazing. I wear my favorite blouse with those shoes I love, a bracelet that reminds me of my goals, and a ring that reminds me of my commitments.

I get dressed not just for the image, but to tell me that I am WORTH the effort. I am motivating myself as I get going in the morning. I don't wake up that way—I have to decide to get there. I am not a morning person. I'm a sleepy morning person. I don't wake up with a purpose; I talk myself into being motivated on purpose. It's not an accident. I don't shame me—Vanity Prayers are about inserting hope into your routine so that you can begin the day with the hope of being AMAZING! They're about arming you with what you need to truly give off the radiant hotness of purpose and honor.

Clients have come to me and said that Vanity Prayers helped them lose weight. Why? Because when you turn off the shame cycle in your own head you will start to be open to what could be. That's what you focus on, and your behavior will fall in line with what you *feel* is possible!

If you tell yourself every day that you are fat, when the brownie is put in front of you, you think, *Well, the damage is already done! I might as well enjoy it!* And you go for the moment of bliss. If you think you can't succeed, you won't—and every time you do something that sabotages your efforts, the shaming, poopy talk in your brain increases. You pull yourself out of the race for what you want. You may blame others for how you feel and what you can't have, but it's *you* who repeats it in your own words and thoughts. What you eat has the power to help your body feel good, and motivation works the same way—you have to get a good diet of inspiration and positive thinking to outweigh the negative, AND your focus has to be in the right place.

No one else can validate you enough to motivate you to go for what you want. In the same way, no one else can hold you back if you want something in the right way.

People post pictures of fancy houses, stacks of money, and dream cars on their fridge. They think money will give them happiness. But that's not what happens: Money just makes you more of what you already are. If you spend more than you have now, you would manage to spend your way through the lottery if you won that. Yet those who work year after year to earn their millions tend to hold on to it. When things come too easily, we tend to take them for granted.

How can you maintain gratitude, motivation, and happiness? Let's go back to eating for a minute. Remember the food pyramid they showed us in school? It shows the healthiest way to eat. It has the fats and sugars in the smallest space at the top, the dairy and meats in the middle, and the grains in the biggest space at the bottom. Maybe you agree with that and maybe you don't. My purpose here isn't to tell you how to eat. After all, I'm not an expert on food—except chocolate, of course.

Every expert recommends eating few or no sugars and no bad oils. Yet we love them so much that when we think of dieting, we focus on what we *can't* have instead of what we *can* have. We deny, shame, and deprive ourselves, and then we wonder why we are discouraged. It's because we are not placing our want in the right place.

You can be happy now. Today. But you have to choose it. As humans, we are prone to place our happiness in the hands of others. Get honest—how many times have you thought something similar to this:

"When they accept me, I'll be happy with me."

"When I have money, I will ..."

"When I get the promotion ..."

"When I am thinner ..."

"I deserve that because I am a good person."

"Life would be easier for me too if I had her brains."

"He was just lucky."

"We could be happy together if you would just ..."

What trapped thinking. You can't be happy *until*. If you put off choosing to be happy, you never will be.

The movie *Cool Runnings* is about the first Jamaican bobsled team. The coach gives one of the athletes who is facing a crisis a profound piece of wisdom: "If you are not enough without it, you will never be enough with it." The Bible tells us to place our hearts on God, not riches. Why is it so hard to focus where we should to get the result we want? Because we want to blame others instead of being responsible for holding ourselves back.

Here's what happens as a result: We spend our energy chasing emotional sugars and oils instead of seeking after the green leafy vegetables and whole grains. We want what feels good or safe now. We would rather beat up on ourselves, repeatedly bemoaning that we can't have what we want, rather than risk failing at the required stretching. We give up happiness with our families, barking at them because of how we feel right now.

When my husband was hit by the bus and I was driving to the hospital, I didn't care if he had put his laundry away where I prefer. When he died in my arms, I didn't care how much money we had in our checking account. When he held me in his arms after finding out that his heart tissue was healed, he didn't care how much love I had around my middle. When our daughter was dying, we didn't care about anything but what we really wanted—to be a family. To love each other. To be living in honor. To have what sacred and precious time we had together.

What we *really* want is not the oils and sugars of life. We want a real connection with ourselves and with others. Yet we spend our energy chasing the fats and sugars. We ask others to feed us the things that will keep us emotionally well fed, and when they don't we are angry with them. Lower your expectations of others and raise your expectations of yourself. When life is so hard that it gets boiled down to what is really important, live with gratitude for what you do have. Focus on what is right, and be responsible when things go wrong. You are in control of you.

After Katelynn died I learned this lesson all the more. It is easier to choose to be really happy when I focus on what is right with my life. I joke that I can't let one thing ruin my life. Don't get me wrong—the death of my daughter was and still is the hardest thing that has happened in my life. When she died, those in our life responded in one of two ways—either with an outpouring of love that I still cherish and offers of service that I can never repay, or with words and actions that were so cruel that they astounded me. They simply couldn't respect what we did or how we responded to Katelynn's life and death. I had thought under the circumstance I should be exempt from others being mean to me. Instead, I learned that life is life. It is unpredictable. I learned the true character of people and I learned my true character and strength. I learned that hard times don't always bring out the best in people, but they do bring out who people truly are.

Our own individual standard of decency may not be the same as those around us. That doesn't mean that we lower our standards. Our world is not a 100 percent one-way trip. It is still full of contrasts. How odd it was that even then, in such a clearly hard situation, some would rush to our side, anxious to help us, while others sought to hurt us and thought of their own comfort instead of our feelings.

Months before Katelynn died I had volunteered to work at a celebration our church was having. My job was to greet and direct the hundreds of visitors. Even though our daughter had died in the interim, I fulfilled my assignment. Yes, I could have called and gotten out of it, but being there made me feel that I was honoring my commitment. I sat smiling in my wheelchair. It felt good to get away for just a few hours to smile at strangers in the midst of planning a funeral. I am really good at applying concealer, so my puffy eyes were hidden behind my smile. It felt really good to do some small service.

As I worked greeting people, a man that knew me began telling other volunteers about Katelynn. A woman came over and told me about her own child who had died years earlier. She began to give me advice, saying, "Don't let others tell you how to grieve." That made sense to me, because others can't really know what you are going through. But something else she said made no sense at all: She told me that it would be years before I could smile again. *What?* By then my kids would be raised and gone! Didn't I love Nathaniel and Ailsa as much as I loved Katelynn? Would I rob them of a happy mom? Would I rob Nathan of the joys of a happy wife? Then she shared her last pearl of wisdom: "I knew the moment that others stopped praying for me." Her grief had totally isolated her. She may have finally arrived at a place where she could tolerate her grief, but she was still angry.

From what she was telling me, she believed that others held her happiness. She was convinced that their prayers sustained her, and that without those prayers she was helpless. (I didn't want those who prayed for us to feel that they had to maintain focus on us.) Where was that woman's focus? On the actions of others? Or on her own connection with God and her own responsibility for her feelings? I don't know her heart, but what I saw was a woman consumed with what others needed to do for her—a woman who, however large her pain and however justifiable her grief, used her grief and pain to place responsibility on other people.

I realized then that the same seeds of hurt lay in me. Was I not painfully aware of how some were treating me? Was I *sooo* aware that they were wrong in doing so? I could wait until I had mourned for a while, until I was "over" some of the hurts, or I could begin to build my own happiness right then.

We all think that when the *ifs* of our lives are removed, when the hurts are gone, when the apologies are given, when the money is attained, then we can finally be happy. I learned from Katelynn's death that my life could never be perfect. I will always miss her. In my life I will never get to see her toddle and fall, and I will never be able to ease her tears with kisses. I won't get to struggle with a late-night homework assignment with her. I won't plan a wedding. I will miss all those things.

One day Winnie, my grandmother figure, sat at our dining room table and told us of the young baby she had lost. Then, wiping her tears, she said, "Here I am crying about a baby that died sixty years ago." I remember that. The loss of Katelynn will always hurt. But I look at Winnie, who had a similar loss. She lived a life of service. She made others happy. She chose to be happy. I could too. Perfect happiness is for heaven. Life is for learning, for honoring what we know is right through what we choose. In focusing my wants on what is really important—by focusing on the juicy greens and wheat germ of life—I can taste happiness many times. I already have.

The funniest nurse we know spoke at Katelynn's funeral. My husband also spoke and shared our conviction of God's hand in our lives. After the flowers died and the trays of food were eaten, people were still people. Some were kind and some were cruel, but through it all we were happy. I have forgiven and lowered my expectations of those that were poopy. It takes time. But I have been given the time to do that.

I am grateful that I get to focus on what is really important every day. Each night I go to sleep, tired from work or play, with the kisses of my family. I take off my makeup and I see my mom's brown eyes and my father's chin and the love of my tummy. I see a beautiful woman full of her own hotness radiating out to impact those around her for good. And every night, looking deep into my soul, I ask myself three questions about my day:

Have I honored myself?

Have I honored those who depend on me?

And have I honored my God?

How do you stay motivated and focused on the good things of life? How do you have happiness and love? Start today. Look yourself in the eye see how amazing you are! Honor your connection with God. See the hotness within you. Do your Vanity Prayers every morning and every night, and one day in the face of all that is hard, ugly, difficult, and discouraging, you will start to see what God sees—the amazing YOU!

See what God sees as your potential and then work, serve, and honor that vision every day. Live with a heart full of gratitude and a mind fed with a diet of the good stuff. Work for what you really want, not what you think you need. You will find that you are stronger and more amazing than you ever thought possible.

Hotness Challenge

You've heard it countless times. Maybe you've even said—or thought—it yourself. I'll be happy *when* I get out of debt. I'll be happy *if* I pass this exam. I'll be happy *when* I get married. I'll be happy *if* my daughter gets the job she applied for. I'll be happy *when* . . . I'll be happy *if* . . .

Just because everybody's saying it doesn't make it right! What sane person would want to put happiness on hold? Bring it on!

There's a fundamental problem with the particular type of thinking I just described. As German inventor Frederick Keonig—best known for his invention of the high-speed printing press—said, "We tend to forget that happiness doesn't come as a result of getting something we don't have, but rather of recognizing and appreciating what we do have." If you're always pinning your hope of happiness on some future event, you'll never be happy. Because as soon as that thing happens— you pay your last bill, you lose forty pounds, you get married, your husband gets the job he's always wanted—there will be a whole new collection of wants and needs, front and center. A whole new collection of reasons to put your happiness on hold. *Again.*

Pooperness.

If you want to be hot, be happy! Think about the people you consider the hottest. They're the ones you want to be around. They don't spend valuable time and energy whining and complaining. They see the good in life. They lift your spirits because *they're* so happy.

Those people don't own the only lot of hotness on the planet, you know. You can be one of them! Russian novelist and philosopher Fyodor Dostoevsky wrote, "Man is fond of counting his troubles, but he does not count his joys. If he counted them up as he ought to, he would see that every lot has enough happiness provided for it."

That's a sophisticated way of saying something very simple: *You can choose to be happy, because there's plenty of happiness to go around.* Abraham Lincoln said it best when he noted, "Most folks are about as happy as they make up their minds to be." Let me guarantee you, there's plenty of happiness and more to go around—and with it, plenty of hotness and more!

Don't place your happiness in the hands of anyone else. Own it! Don't wait for *ifs* to be removed, apologies to be given, hurts to be eased, money to be attained. Be happy *right now*. Here's a good way to start:

1. Be happy *right now* by focusing on what's right in your life. Don't know exactly what that is? Don't let another minute go by without figuring it out! Take out your trusty notebook. Start writing. List the things that are really, truly good and right in your life right now. *Not* the things you *hope for* but the things that are right this very minute.

2. Now put your list to work! You're getting expert at Vanity Prayers, and that's a great place to focus on what's right in your life. Every day for the next week, include a different

item from your list in each of your Vanity Prayers, day and night. Express sincere gratitude as you focus on one of the things that's right in your life.

3.   Don't keep it to yourself. At least once a day for the next week, share with someone else how grateful you are for one of the things that's right in your life.

4.   No matter what's going on in your life at any given moment, *smile*. That's not just a good idea—there's *science* behind it. According to Dr. Dale Anderson—for five decades a family physician, board-certified surgeon, and board-certified emergency physician—smiling causes the brain to release endorphins, natural chemicals with a structure similar to morphine that act as "natural uppers" in the body. In addition to enhancing health and relieving pain, they are known as the "happy chemicals" because—as the name implies—they bring on a burst of happiness. According to Dr. Anderson (and many others), the quickest way to bring on the endorphins is to simply *smile*. It's the fastest and easiest way to change your brain chemistry—and with it, your outlook on life. And you're not the only one who benefits: smiles are contagious. Everyone who sees your smile will be tempted to do the same!

There. Notice an increase in your hotness? Reflect on that and jot down some notes. And whenever one of the boogie men creeps in and starts spreading gloom and despair (and you *know* they will), stop what you're doing. Take a deep breath. Remember the things that are right in your life right this minute. And *smile* like you mean it.

Chapter Fifteen

——————— 🔥 ———————

TAG, YOU'RE IT
SPREAD THE HOTNESS

MOTHER TERESA SAID, "When people leave you, they should be better and happier." Everything we do impacts others. Even if we feel alone, we aren't. Think about it: If you retreat and withdraw to your grumpy corner, others will wonder why. And if you live in your grumpy corner all the time, you rob those who love you and could love you from getting to know you. You are robbing the world of you!

Giving others compliments is easy to do when you stop berating yourself. You suddenly can see what is right with the world instead of seeing its flaws. One time we were walking up a mountain to see some cyclists in the Tour of Utah; we wanted to cheer them on at their next station. As we walked, I saw a lady with a truckload of boys; all of them were dressed in their best. I looked at her and said, "You are the best-dressed lady on this mountain!" She replied, "Oh, you made my day!" I didn't stop and give her my card, letting her know that I was a professional makeup artist, image consultant, and kind of a kick-butt, awesome expert on such matters, and she should be thankful I noticed her and commented on it. I just smiled and wished her a great day.

My son turned to me and said, "Mom, you always do that."

"Do what?" I asked.

His reply was precious to me, proving the point that we never know what and who we are teaching: "You always make other people's day. You make people happy."

One great thing about getting older is that people no longer erroneously assume that I haven't yet experienced hardship. But they do seem to erroneously think that if I *had*, I wouldn't be so cheerful! Being happy is a choice. When you choose it for you, you get to share it with your children, your spouse, and even random strangers.

Among everything I have accomplished in my life and all the things I expect to accomplish, nothing is more important than those whose lives I have really impacted. I have impacted no one more than my own children—not even my husband, because he was already impressive and awesome when I married him. I did not make him the man he is. We have helped each other in our life and careers, but I am talking about *character*. He already had his amazing character when he married me.

My children are my greatest work. I have been entrusted to love them and to teach them in a day and a culture when the job of being a mother is generally looked down upon. Once, before speaking at a large conference, the person introducing me wanted to trim my bio; that was fine, but the part they wanted to cut was about my being a wife and mom. I suggested that the audience would be comprised of many wives and mothers and that taking out other titles would be better. After that experience I always wrote in my bio that "among all my accomplishments, I am most proud that my husband and children currently like me."

We feel so sad for Scrooge in *A Christmas Carol* because he focuses on things instead of people. When he finally chooses to turn his focus from getting to giving, we celebrate. It's a classic that was written well more than a century ago . . . it looks like human character has been struggling with this for some time!

The applause life gives me is not who I am—and it definitely is not what is most important. We are not our degrees, our titles, or our accomplishments. These are just things we have done. For good or bad, the events of our life do not define us. Would you rather have your tombstone celebrate you as a business tycoon or as a beloved wife and mother?

When a woman introduces herself and says she is "just a mom," I get very verbal: "There is never *just a mom*! When you first puked in a toilet you knew this would change your life. When that baby was first placed in your arms—regardless of whether you're the one who gave birth—you knew you would not only die for that child, but you would change your whole life for the welfare and care of that child. And for months when that child wakes you in the middle of the night—an act that would get a college roommate slaughtered!—you go to that child's bed with love and exhaustion, and you do it day after day! You will even choose for that child to hate you if it teaches the child. You are not *just a mom*—they can't hire people to love!"

Whenever I go on a tirade like this, the poor recipient is usually wide-eyed, wondering what drugs I am taking. Sometimes she is teary-eyed as well. But I mean every single word of it. I would never tear myself down by saying I am *just a mom*, and I can't let anyone else belittle themselves that way either. Sometimes you need to give others a Vanity Prayer of their own!

I have always worked, but I have also always considered myself a stay-at-home mother. I was always home with my children. By the time I finished putting my hubby through law school, Nathaniel was almost three and Ailsa was six months old. I chose to place my focus on raising my children, though I did do some work. Maintaining my SeneGence and image businesses took about two hours a day of focused work; I got all fancied up when I wanted to. Mostly, I crafted, play-grouped, and went on midmorning walks to look for ladybugs. I was not a suppressed woman being kept at home. I felt great pride in the daily work of family and home. For me it was an "empowered" time of my womanhood.

Had events of my life been different, I would have been perfectly content to be a full-time stay-at-home mom who never stood on a stage. I consider it a blessing that my husband's income and the residual income of my business has allowed me the comfort of doing what I choose. As I say that, it is not my intention to hurt the hearts of women who long to be home and can't be for financial reasons. I also realize that not all women want to stay at home.

I don't know where you fall on that spectrum, but I do know one thing: Wherever you are, even if it's not quite where you'd like to be, you have the chance to choose happiness. To choose fulfillment. To choose to impact those around you in a meaningful way. And as you choose those things, you will also choose to become the hottie you are, inside *and* out!

Be it a new day, a course of life, or business, we all have to show up to serve. To honor our purpose. We don't get to predict the outcome but we can choose to honor what we know to be our best. When I speak to business people, I explain that when we look at the client with a dollar amount in our head, we are treating them like fresh meat; we can't really serve them if we don't see them. We need to build a relationship of trust to be honored with the sale.

When you start your day, don't look at the tasks ahead of you as things that have to be done. Instead, look at what could be and what is possible, and choose to represent yourself at your best so you can honor that day, the people in it, and yourself. You can't boil down your value to a dress size, an income amount, or even a specific outcome. Your value is based on honoring what you can be and what you can do. Each of us, no matter how hard or humble our circumstances, can work to honor our day. That sort of commitment starts with you—with what you think is possible.

Each of us has to do the work that leads to the results we want. If we do that, consistently, every day, in the end we will be surprised—in awe, really—of where we end up. Stunning yourself by surpassing what you thought possible is far better than getting to a goal dress size or dollar amount.

In 2005 we were living in Hyattsville, Maryland, in the cheapest housing I could find that wasn't literally in the hood. It was right next to the hood. My hubby had a *non*paid internship with the Federal Court of Appeals in Washington, DC. We were living off what my business brought in, along with a prayer. This was not the kind of neighborhood that organized mommy time at the park.

The one time I had to go to the doctor, the office was so unsanitary that I was concerned my three-year-old son would catch something from the upholstery. I held my baby girl tightly in my arms. Keep in mind I am the kind of mom that if the pacifier falls out I pick it up, plop it in my mouth, sanitize it with my mommy saliva, and give it back to the baby. But had a binky fallen out on this floor, I would have backed away and left it as a casualty of war. It was that bad. The only assurance I had that the doctor hadn't given me anything that would make me high was a bullet-pocked sign on the front door saying there were no painkillers in the building. It was all very comforting.

Our high-rise had no playground, but it did have lots of cockroaches. I found it more comforting to walk my trash out to the far Dumpster than to throw it down the conveniently located trash chute, where I would be greeted by robust roaches awaiting my contribution. Whenever I walked to the grocery store I was verbally threatened, as my hip condition had resulted in a very pronounced limp. I often felt like the lame wildebeest among a pack of pacing lions. Until one day.

A group of men managed a very busy business just outside our building that attracted a lot of car traffic. As there was no playground, the kids all played at the far end of the parking lot. Boys ranging in age from eight to twelve played football with the one ball they had. My son was anxious to join them—but because he was so much younger than the rest of the boys, I hesitated.

One day his exuberance earned him an invitation from the group of regulars. I told the boys that I appreciated their kindness and would make cookies the day they played with him. They looked at me like I was from a different planet. I kinda was. But there I was, carrying my famous homemade chocolate chip cookies in one hand and my baby, Ailsa, in my other, while the boys played football in the parking lot.

The boys created a special position for my son on the team; they called it "baby drop-back." I enjoyed watching them play from a position where I could slow oncoming cars. One of the businessmen, hearing that I had chocolate chip cookies, came over and asked if he could have one. Of course, I told him. He took the entire plate. Later I found it outside my apartment door on the second floor.

My son became a welcome addition to Denzel, Mohamed, Elijah, and Chris. He was a member of their football team, and I was making a lot of cookies. Then came the day that changed everything.

That day, a car in the parking lot a car was going far too fast. Moving as quickly as could, I began to yell—the car was headed straight toward where my young son was playing. Suddenly one of the gentlemen who hung out in the parking lot stepped in front of the car; it screeched to a halt. Out of breath, I arrived just in time to hear the driver apologize profusely to my new hero. I thanked the man who had risked his own safety to stop a careless driver. As I gathered up my son, waiting for my pounding heart to slow, I heard him say, "You're welcome, Mrs. Greene."

When I told my mother this story, she was unnerved to find that he knew my name. But he had known my name the moment our U-Haul truck drove up. After the incident in the parking lot, he often looked in on me. Once he even pulled out a large roll of money, explaining to me that he was a businessman and could help me with anything I needed—Food? Rent? Diapers? Anything? I thanked him for his kindness and made sure that cookies always found their way to his place of business.

From then on as I walked to the grocery store, the men who had previously yelled out to me became silent. Instead, they offered to carry my groceries. I was under the protection of the neighborhood "businessman."

The boys started coming over to our apartment right after school. I instituted a homework time. We read together. We made mini pizzas, and they eagerly declared that I was "a great cooker." When the weather was bad, they threw the ball around our apartment as I sat on the couch feeding my baby. They asked me questions. As I told them about running through open fields and showed them pictures of my hikes in Alaska and the Grand Canyon, they made art and entertained my son.

I finally realized with some sadness that what attracted them to us was not the food—it was the love that came with it. My apartment represented not only a slice of good old suburbia, but a home filled with kind words. I called them—as I call all young people—"Awesome." ("Hey, Awesome, what's up?") They loved it when Mr. Greene came home, and they laughed when he kissed me. Their homes didn't have a mom and a dad; their stories were common for that neighborhood, but they were heartbreaking to me.

One day all the boys were watching *The Incredibles* when a woman's tirade of anger, bad language, and crudity came streaming through the open window. My boys looked at me; it was clear they were humiliated. My son looked toward the window in shock. Asking one of the boys to close the window and another to pause the video, I asked why they were so embarrassed by the woman's behavior. Was she their mom? No. Their aunt? No. Then why were they so embarrassed? She didn't represent them, and they were not responsible for her actions.

They finally told me that because her skin color and theirs was the same, her behavior put them down. Tears filling my eyes, I told the boys what was in my heart. I told them that skin color didn't hold them, bind them, or dictate what could be theirs. I explained that because someone else had my same color of skin didn't mean I was held by that. I told them that all of us—them, the crazy lady outside the window, my son, and I—were all children of God. And I testified that that fact alone told them more than anything about what was possible for them. I reminded them that others had escaped the hood and improved the world. I told them that others had done great things with their lives, and I expressed the belief that they would too.

They looked at me as if I had just offered them the rarest and most delicious dessert in all the world.

"Why do people worry about children in the hood?" I asked them. They answered quickly—drugs, sex, other things I didn't want my son to hear. He was sitting in the lap of one of the boys, who was rubbing his foot tenderly. What they saw as possible for their life was what they saw.

I told them of where I came from—a place where the streets had trees, where most moms stayed home and most kids went to college. I explained that we always assumed we would go to college because that's what the other kids did. "Where you come from, boys, does not decide where you will go in life," I explained. "What you THINK is possible is where you will go." I challenged them to see life as possible—to see past the "hood," to be like those who had left the hood and been forces of good.

We talked for a long time that day. We talked of schooling, of making good choices. We talked about what kinds of choices trapped us and what kinds of choices offered a better life. By the time the conversation ended, we were all sitting together on the couch. Suddenly Mohamed hugged me and said, "Mrs. Greene, someday I am going to show up at your door and thank you for all of your kindness."

Hugging him back, I said, "Mohamed, I will plan on it."

Mohamed would be nineteen now. I hope he has chosen to be awesome and . . . well, incredible. Those boys all have my toll-free business number. That number will never change, just in case one of my boys decides to call.

My hope for those boys—the hope we all have for those who have so much less yet have the same potential any of us do—is that I somehow reached into their hearts and gave them a taste of the love of God for them. I hope I gave them a dose of dreams to keep their fire burning. I hope that the kindness they showed me and my son has not been crushed by the hardness of their environment. I hope that they will see beyond their surroundings and choose to be the men they can be.

I hold that same hope for you. I hope that in sharing some of my story I will help you look beyond what you know right here, right now, and that you will choose to be awesome, amazing, and HOT. Share it, be it, and realize that the spark you are feeling is God saying that you are enough, that you are worth it, and that He will be there to help you. Are you ready to be stunned with who you really are? Just ask Him, and get to work in embracing your inner hotness!

Hotness Challenge

The hottest people I know all have one thing in common: They focus on *people*, not *things*. They honor their purpose. Their priority isn't the biggest house, the fastest car, the boat or the snowmobile or the European vacation. It's the chance to impact someone else— the opportunity to make a difference in someone's life. They don't get their kicks from a two-carat diamond solitaire; they get their kicks from helping someone else do or feel something really great. When all is said and done, they yearn to make a difference in the life of someone else. They hope to leave this world a richer place for having been here.

There are many ways to make an impact, and many of them require an impressive bank account. But there's at least one that won't cost you a penny. It's so simple that you can do it numerous times a day without making the slightest dent in your own time, energy, or resources. Yet its impact can be amazing. In fact, it can be the catalyst that can change someone else for the better.

What is it?

A compliment.
Try it now:

1. At least three times a day for the next week, give someone you meet a compliment.

2. Your compliment needs to be sincere and genuine. So what if the woman next to you in the grocery store line is not a raving beauty? Compliment her on the color of her eyes. The cute jacket she's wearing. The kind way she dealt with the grouchy customer in front of her. The way her smile cheered you up even though the weather outside is dismal. You get the idea.

3. Remember to *smile* when you dish out your compliments. Author Leo F. Buscaglia reminds us, "Too often we underestimate the power of a touch, a smile, a kind word, a listening ear, an honest compliment, or the smallest act of caring, all of which have the potential to turn a life around."

Now that you have finished your makeover, make this last behavior—the bestowal of compliments—a habit. Reflect on how much your hotness has increased, where you are now compared to where you were the day you first picked up this book. Remember that what you think is possible is where you will go . . . so go all the way! And while you're at it, take others with you by spreading the hotness!

Acknowledgments

IN 2008 I gave a speech to a group of about four hundred young girls, ranging in age from twelve to eighteen, and their volunteer youth leaders. One of those volunteers was Angela Eschler. After I spoke to the girls about their potential, how amazing they were, and to be promise-keepers to themselves and God, Angela said I should write a book. I laughed! How funny—me, write a book! Ha! I had a very good list of reasons why I shouldn't write a book. After all, I write like I talk—in run-on-and-on sentences. Also, who would want to buy a book I wrote? I was unknown, living in the suburbs, driving a minivan, and loving life. If I'd had a LinkedIn profile it would have listed childrearing, potty training, scrapbooking, home decorating, and eating chocolate as my main pursuits. My professional days were behind me and I was savoring motherhood.

I didn't recognize a possible talent for sharing my experiences in a meaningful way. I didn't remember getting As in creative writing, or, when I did, think that would have qualified me to write a book. Nor did the years of telling people what I thought about beauty, self-esteem, confidence, marriage, and happiness. What I did feel at the idea of writing a book was fear—and so I laughed. I laughed loudly at anyone and everyone who said I should write it. How crazy would that be!! Angela kept coming around, asking me—during what I call our "adventure years"—if I was keeping a journal. To which my answer was, "Yes . . . for my own private personal use!"

Then there was Katelynn. She changed me; she changed everyone who knew her. I was blessed to be her mom. I was blessed to be Nathaniel's and Ailsa's mom. Did they not deserve an example—a mom who was doing her best and using the time and talents given her? The answer scared me, but after burying a child, what was fear? It was only an emotion. What had I taught my clients, what did I stand for, what would I say to my children? When everything is stripped away in grief, you either collapse into the loss that yanks at you, or you find your footing and awaken to your strength. It's not just that I was a survivor. I had been given new perspective—something to share. I saw little snippets of my life differently in my new clarity, and I saw myself clearly: I was not my fears, not my self-described limitations, but a woman who had done and overcome great things already to be a well-adjusted and happily-not-insane adult. Shouldn't I share how I'd done that? I could see that what I knew about life was a gift, and all gifts or talents are to be shared. The teenage girl with no talents had a talent after all.

To my kids, Nathaniel, Ailsa, and Katelynn—thank you for sharing your mom. It probably feels unfair that your mom has to run a business, speak, and write a book, but I can see you learning good things from all of that too.

One day as I was talking to my son about a struggle he was having, I started giving him the age-appropriate/male version of Vanity Prayers. He asked me where I had learned this stuff. I told him that's what I do when I am gone speaking or teaching my "stuff." He looked at me like he was amazed that his mom was that smart—the same look he gives me when I make his favorite meal on a tough day—and said, "Mom, this is great stuff; you should tell more people!" I am trying, son. Thank you for believing in your crazy, talks-too-much mom. And to Ailsa, who secured my pinky-promise that I would give her the first book, who, every night when I tuck her in, asks me what my favorite part of the day was. Invariably it is being a mom to her and her brother. And to my Katelynn, my baby pearl, I'm working to live up to who you showed me I truly am. Kids are my greatest contribution to the world.

I am equally honored to be the wife of Nathan Greene. A man who prizes routine and who, for some mysterious reason, still likes me and loves me too!—two things that I feel blessed for daily. Of course, I am an amazing wife. How could he resist all this Hotness??!

I thank my family for the late nights that I escaped to the office to write, laughing and crying as I did so. They had some subpar meals so that I could get my writing in.

I want to thank my parents, who live in our basement. My mother's body is broken with MS, but her support and encouragement . . . well, you know those kids who sing on *American Idol* who are, well, not so . . . ? My mom gave me that kind of encouragement. My parents would buy all my book copies had they the money, just to make me feel good about my efforts. Fortunately they won't have to. All nine of my best friends have promised to buy a book.

My friends, thank you for still being there when I call. Inviting me to lunch. Calling me. Encouraging me. Cynthia, Stacey, Chelsea, Raquel, Candice, Candas, Taryn, Gail, and Jessica, thank you for dropping things to come stand by me when we said good-bye to Katelynn and for standing by me when I have neglected our friendship to be living at full speed. I am blessed with amazing women as my friends.

I didn't let anyone read the book in the beginning stages; only small parts were shared. I wanted it to pass my test first. It had to be the best I could do. Then I turned it over to Angela and her amazing team at Eschler Editing. Thank you to Sabine, Kathy, Michele, and Ben (book design) for reining in my ADD and telling me where I needed to fix this or that. Kinda hated it at times. But the reader thanks you for fixing my grammar. When Mr. Greene read it, he said, "It's you with good grammar!" Thank you for pushing me to my full hotness as a writer. And, Angela—thank you for seeing in me what I thought was so hilarious. Me . . . write a book!! Crazy, huh?

This may seem odd, but I also want to thank the people who have been poopy—the authors of angry letters when I chose not to respond to Katelynn's passing with anger or resentment. The tension in our conversations, and the purposeful misinterpretation of what I said and did, revealed to me that, in spite of opposition, I had to shine. I wanted to keep a connection with you, but you wouldn't let me be me, and that is not hot. I choose to live at full awesomeness. I am here when you are ready to join me.

In church one day the cover design of the book came to me. I was so excited that my love had to remind me to be quiet. Thank you to Kent of Worth Designing for taking my ideas and making them real and so amazingly hot!!

And Stonebridge Printing has done everything from my business cards to . . . well, my book! They offered amazing customer service even when I was a small client. Thank you, Jennifer and Jill!

I want to thank, above all, my Savior Jesus Christ, for making me more than I thought possible. Thank you for giving me your strength. I am going to have to keep on borrowing your light. Thank you for trusting me with these words, gifts, talents, and with my precious children and hubby. All I have that is good is from God. These days, all that I have that is poopy . . . I did that myself, and I am working on it.

Thank you to you, the reader, for parting with your time. I hope that your heart and mind are inspired on your path to your own extreme hotness!

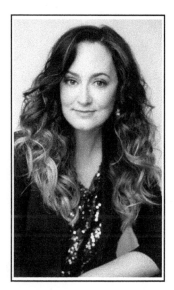

About the Author

A flannel-clad member of the setup crew for her dad's mobile-home-moving company, Leta Greene was raised in what she calls two extremes: truck stops and Provo, Utah. Not exactly spots that belched up beauty tips. So how did a shy tomboy with her share of scars become a confident beauty expert?

Here's a clue: it didn't involve a traditional makeover, or even much makeup! She discovered the secret to lasting beauty—and it worked despite all the scars and truck stops. Now she works tirelessly to share that secret, both as the founder of Glamour Connection®, an image consulting company, and as one of the most influential women of SeneGence International.

Featured on major TV stations as a beauty expert, Leta speaks on more than just beauty—she talks about life in a way that makes you laugh your heart out! She's in demand as a trainer and motivator, but after just a few minutes you'll realize she communicates far more than words.

What does this talented woman consider her most important accomplishment? "Easy!" she laughs, "my husband and children still like me!" You can find Leta—and access her beauty blog to get more detailed tips (and visual aids) for your hottest look—at yourglamourconnection.com and letagreene.com.

CPSIA information can be obtained
at www.ICGtesting.com
Printed in the USA
BVHW040225230821
615006BV00014B/1108